DATE DUE

GAYLORD   #3522PI   Printed in USA

D1469061

THE BODY HUNTERS

Also by Sonia Shah

Crude: The Story of Oil

THE BODY HUNTERS

Testing New Drugs on the World's Poorest Patients

SONIA SHAH

THE NEW PRESS

NEW YORK
LONDON

Requests for permission to reproduce selections from this book should be
mailed to: Permissions Department, The New Press, 38 Greene Street,
New York, NY 10013.

Published in the United States by The New Press, New York, 2006
Distributed by W. W. Norton & Company, Inc., New York

LIBRARY OF CONGRESS CATALOGING-IN-PUBLICATION DATA

Shah, Sonia.
    The body hunters : testing new drugs on the world's poorest patients /
Sonia Shah.
       p. cm.
    Includes bibliographical references and index.
    ISBN-13: 978-1-56584-912-9 (hc.)
    ISBN-10: 1-56584-912-4 (hc.)
    1. Pharmaceutical policy—Developing countries.   2. Pharmaceutical
industry—Corrupt   practices—Developing   countries.   3. Drugs—
Prescribing—Developing countries.   4. Drug utilization—Developing
countries.   5. Medical ethics.   I. Title.

    RA401.D44S53   2006
    362.17'82—dc22   2005058394

The New Press was established in 1990 as a not-for-profit alternative to
the large, commercial publishing houses currently dominating the book
publishing industry. The New Press operates in the public interest rather
than for private gain, and is committed to publishing, in innovative ways,
works of educational, cultural, and community value that are often
deemed insufficiently profitable.

www.thenewpress.com

Composition by Westchester Book Composition
This book was set in Palatino

Printed in the United States of America

10 9 8 7 6 5 4 3 2 1

Contents

Foreword

JOHN LE CARRÉ

This book is an act of courage on the part of its author and its publishers. Ever since I wrote *The Constant Gardener*, I have received approaches, and sometimes complete typescripts, from investigative writers determined to lift the veil on the darker side of the world's most profitable trade: the pharmaceutical industry. Where a proposed book seemed to have merit, and was not weighed down with mountains of medical jargon, I passed the word to literary agents and publishers' readers. Yet not one of the authors, so far as I was ever aware, saw his project realized. And if, months later, I delicately inquired why not, the answer, however wrapped up, was always the same: too risky.

And you might find it comic or outrageous or, if you are of my mind-set, illustrative of the stranglehold of unrestricted corporate power that the topic that is closest to all our lives, and closest to the concerns and responsibilities that we feel for one another, should be deemed too risky for public debate.

You might also find it outrageous that our treasured legal system, originally designed to protect our freedoms, should be the instrument of their suppression. Yet such is the reputation of the gunslinging lawyers of Big Pharma, so unlimited the industry's wealth, so vast its reach into politics, the media, and the very heart of the medical profession and the bureaucracy that sustains it, that publishers have good reason to believe that, in picking a fight with Big Pharma, they are committing their company to a five-star lawsuit, countless hours of office time, disenchanted stockholders, and copies pulped before they reach the stores.

Yet, little by little, the veil is indeed being lifted. The outsourcing of clinical trials to countries where sick people are so poor they are ready to sign up to anything, whether or not they can read what's on the consent form, is now public knowledge. The tendency of Big Pharma to promote phantom, or at best speculative, maladies and then supply the cure for them, is now public knowledge.

The corrupt recruitment of large numbers of doctors in general practice and teaching hospitals to prescribe a particular medical project is now public knowledge

The corrupt recruitment of large numbers of doctors in general practice and teaching hospitals to prescribe a particular medical product is now public knowledge.

The ever-growing list of dangerously under-tested products that have been wished upon the public by supposedly impartial government bodies is public knowledge, as are the links between members of such bodies and the pharmaceutical companies that manufactured them.

It is also public knowledge, since they themselves have owned to it, that learned medical journals of supposed integrity have carried glowing accounts of this or that pharmaceutical product, only to discover they were written not by the august Professor of Something who has put his name to them but by their manufacturers.

But perhaps the worst of Big Pharma's many sins is its persistent encroachment, by means of a combination of lavish sponsorship and moral blackmail, on the integrity of biomedical research at every level, with the consequent ever-growing scarcity of unbought medical minds.

Using clear, accessible language and carefully annotated case histories, Sonia Shah has struck a blow for all who dream of har-

nessing the huge power for good that is invested in the pharmaceutical industry, of seeing its products made available to those
who most need them, and of curtailing the greed that drives its
worst practices.

Cornwall, England
February 2006

Preface

"The blood of those who will die if biomedical research is not pursued will be upon the hands of those who don't do it."

—Joshua Lederberg, PhD, Nobel laureate[1]

"I mean, shit, we learn by climbing over the bodies of humans."

—Murray Gardner, MD, University of California HIV researcher[2]

"Field trials are indispensable. . . . If, in major medical dilemmas, the alternative is to pay the cost of perpetual uncertainty, have we really any choice?"

—Donald Frederickson, MD, former National Institutes of Health (NIH) director[3]

My life and the lives of some of my closest relatives continue thanks to the interventions of modern medicine, a scientific art that has marched forward in fits and starts on a bedrock of clinical research. The drugs that enabled me to survive an emergency cesarean section, those that allow my son to breathe despite allergic asthma, the other ones that correct a hormonal deficit in my mother have been administered to us with success and confidence in part because they've been tested in hundreds and perhaps thousands of human subjects in experimental trials. Not only that: these successful drugs emerge from a slurry of countless other failed drugs, each of which was also tested on scores of warm bodies, some of which may have been harmed by their shortcomings.

There's nothing terrible about the truth that medical research imposes burdens. But generally speaking, we don't like to know it. We don't like to see it. The very notion of experimenting upon humans sounds sinister. And yet, if anything, we only want ever more drugs to help or enhance us, and more data to assure our trembling selves of their safety and effectiveness. The response to these contradictory desires has been the same since the mid-1800s, when scientists hell-bent on dissecting animals skirted the outcries of British antivivisectionists by cloaking their slicing in secrecy. Today, savvy drugmakers loudly publicize new medical products, but conduct the required experimentation quietly. And so, while we exult in, bicker over, and complain about the products of medical research—how much do the drugs cost? who pays? what are the side effects?—the vast business of percolating new drugs burrows underground.

If the history of human experimentation tells us anything, from the bloody vivisections of the first millennium to the Tuskegee Syphilis Study, it is that the potential for abuse will fall heaviest on the poorest and most powerless among us.

The trend within the drug industry to conduct their experimental drug trials in poor countries is, as yet, in its infancy. But it is growing fast. Major drugmakers such as GlaxoSmithKline, Wyeth and Merck—already conducting between 30 and 50 percent of their experiments outside the United States and Western Europe—plan to step up the number of their foreign trials by up to 67 percent by 2006, according to *USA Today*. And while armies of clinical investigators in the United States shrink, dropping by 11 percent between 2001 and 2003, those abroad fatten, increasing by 8 percent over the same period, according to a 2005 study by the Tufts Center for Drug Development. "The outsourcing of drug research is beginning to accelerate," reported the *Washington Post* in May 2005.[4]

And all the pressures on the profit-driven industry, pushing it toward speed and ever-lower costs; Americans' contradictory love of new drugs and skittishness about participating in the experiments that make them possible; the increasing desperation of hordes of patients in developing countries deprived access to useful medicines; and the immediate financial needs of the cash-strapped public hospitals and clinics meant to serve them suggest the trend will only grow over the coming years. Many leaders in developing countries, faced with crumbling facilities, minuscule budgets, and towering health crises make arrangements for more industry trials, not fewer.

It is a trend that cries out for public review. That's because the consequences of the multinational drug industry's trek into the developing world go far beyond the fates of the patients roped into their trials and then discarded afterward. After all, many will be helped, at least for the brief moments of their participation, and that is not insignificant.

More troubling are the potential implications for health care in poor countries. As clinical trials become an ever-larger cash cow for strapped hospitals and clinics, a larger portion of scarce resources gets diverted away from providing care. In many countries governments have stoked the trend by tightening up patent laws, easing ethics reviews of experiments, and converting medical record keeping into industry-friendly English. Nurses, doctors, and other clinicians already overwhelmed with needy patients find themselves with even less time for healing when institutional priorities shift from treating the ill to experimenting upon them for drug companies. And whether it is a quickie experiment or a well-intentioned study, if ethical oversight is shoddy or patient subjects uncomprehending of its purposes, the mistrust engendered runs deep, contaminating all of Western medicine's offerings, including life-saving vaccines and medicines.

The business of experimentation in developing countries intensifies the pressure to crack open these markets for the sales of new brand-name drugs too, by adding the quid pro quo demands of local clinicians and government officials proffering their patients as experimental fodder. Pfizer, Eli Lilly, GlaxoSmithKline, and other drug giants jostle at the borders of India, Brazil, Russia, and China, foreseeing huge markets for their cholesterol-lowering, antidepressant, and erectile-dsyfunction-alleviating blockbusters. The industry's philosophy of equating medical innovation with "new products" is especially pernicious in places where simpler solutions have yet to be attempted. While innovative approaches to the health dilemmas posed by the lack of clean water and safe food, for example, are needed, the answer does not lie in new brand-name drugs. And even when new products are indeed what are most needed, from new malaria drugs to cures for sleeping sickness, those that aid the poorest are generally of little interest to drug companies, which commit themselves to the financial needs of their investors. The more likely result will be a drug-marinated class of rich alongside a meds-famished poor. In that case, brand-name drug sales in poor countries will worsen inequality, not correct it. And as has been well documented, inequality itself worsens the health of the have-nots even more.

Finally, we need to open up the debate over the very idea of using human bodies as experimental matter. For some, performing the work of an experimental test subject is the same as, say, taking a job in a factory. But for many others, industry trials in poor countries offer an impossible choice—be experimented on or die for lack of medicine—that undermines human rights. In the streets of Lagos and the halls of international AIDS conferences, people from developing countries are condemning Western scientists' use of them as guinea pigs. The body hunters disregard the growing outcry at their peril.

1

Clinical Trials Go Global

On a dull October day in 2003 a clutch of physicians and scientists meet in a windowless conference room in the basement of a Washington, DC, hotel. John Wurzlemann, MD, flashes a photograph of modern-day Poland on a white screen to a handful of his colleagues. A generic urban scene, with glittering steel-and-glass buildings encircled by cement sidewalks appears. Wurzlemann, a rumpled, soft-spoken man, grins ruefully. "Most of Poland does not look like this," he notes, in a deep scratchy voice. "Most of it looks like how it looked in 1939," during the Nazi and Soviet invasions. "My father went to Poland ten years ago, and he said nothing had changed since the 1930s. Everything just got older."

And sicker. Just how sick Eastern Europeans have become was the topic of Wurzlemann's late-afternoon lecture that day. Broke, malnourished, and fatally enamored of cigarettes, Eastern Europeans were dropping dead in scores, he told the crowd. While in the United States deaths from cardiovascular disease had been falling steadily since the 1960s, in Eastern Europe cardiovascular disease had mushroomed to epidemic proportions and killed people far more rapidly.[1] Wurzlemann was nothing if not blunt. "Disease for disease," he said, "they are more likely to die."

Wurzlemann moved quickly through his PowerPoint presentation, offering up a deluge of discomfiting facts and figures. "Hungary has the highest rate of cervical cancer mortality.... Breast cancer rates are higher.... Cancer mortality among men in Poland is the highest in Eastern Europe.... Suicide rates are a lot higher."

He paused briefly for a slide showing a map of Europe, which had blood-red marks indicating the death rate from all causes. "What it shows," Wurzlemann said, as the audience gazed on silently, "is that as you go east, people die in increasing waves." Indeed, it looked as if a bottle of red ink had been spilled over the map of Russia. The stain had spread over all of Eastern Europe too, but France, Italy, and Spain were nearly pristine, marred by a scant few speckles. National borders marked the difference between life and death, drawn in whispery black lines.

The Eastern Europeans were ailing not only because their air was polluted, their food less abundant, and their water dirtier, Wurzlemann said. The amount of money the Polish government coughed up to provide health care to each of its citizens was about one-fourth the sum typical in Western Europe. Such paltry investments typified the region. As a result, preventive techniques, early diagnostic methods, and medical treatments that had transformed killer diseases into manageable chronic illnesses and better in the West were as rare as those shiny skyscrapers. Wurzlemann didn't mention it, but the same could be said for much of the rest of the world too, where well over half of humanity has been brutally left behind in the quest for good health and longevity.

Wurzlemann took a deep breath and turned to his expectant audience. He himself had enjoyed the benefits of the West's good health, wealth, and education, although two generations before him had hailed from ailing Poland and Russia. He grinned and softly muttered, almost to himself: "It is really upsetting, frankly." Then he briskly returned to his presentation and its scripted points.[2]

The speakers who followed Wurzlemann offered their own tales of woe from Latin America, Asia, and South Africa. Ordinarily, a group of physicians confronted with such information would respond with any number of suggestions aimed at alleviating the burden of misery. Might more health care training help? Cheaper drugs? More research into disease etiology? Better diagnostic techniques? But neither Wurzlemann nor the other speakers had traveled to Washington, DC, that day to persuade their colleagues to help the impoverished sick of the developing world, at least not in the standard way that doctors generally try to help patients.

They had gathered because multinational drug companies like Pfizer, Eli Lilly, and Merck had a business problem. Industry labs were bursting with spanking new compounds and insight into which human tissues to aim them at, courtesy of new techniques first pioneered by genetic engineers and biotechnologists in the 1970s. "There are more investigational new drugs, more experimental treatments today . . . than ever before," former Food and Drug Administration commissioner Mark McClellan exulted before a meeting of industry researchers in 2003.[3] But just as the biotech revolution took off, the pipeline turning those new compounds into sellable products had started to clog. Proving new drugs worked in humans, as required by the FDA, had become a spectacularly complex, expensive, and time-consuming endeavor, a constant cause for complaints from industry analysts and investigators. Clinical trials were a "vast canyon" that eviscerated new drugs; a veritable "valley of death," they said.[4] "Large trials have become the norm," bemoaned another. "All professionals taking part are now reconciled to the idea that such trials will take forever and will cost the earth."[5]

According to CenterWatch, a publisher specializing in the clinical research industry, in order to launch a single drug a company has to convince more than 4,000 patients to undergo 141 medical procedures each in more than 65 separate trials. First come the small Phase 1 studies that test a new drug's safety; then the slightly larger Phase 2 studies that look for hints of effectiveness, and finally the extensive Phase 3 studies that aim to prove a drug's effectiveness with statistical certainty. More than 100,000 people have to be enticed to call in for initial screenings for such trials, as only a fraction show up for their appointments, and of these only a fraction would be medically eligible.[6] With the expense of finding and retaining a single test subject for a clinical trial running to at least $1,500, and with some 90 percent of the drugs entering clinical trials failing to garner FDA approval anyway, minimizing the cost and length of clinical trials had become crucial to corporate salubrity.[7]

And yet, in the United States at least, enlisting sufficient numbers of trial volunteers is difficult, to say the least. Back in 1954, Americans offered their children as human guinea pigs by the millions for Jonas Salk's experimental polio vaccine. When the results of that massive trial were released, radio announcers blasted the news. Church bells clanged. Traffic snarled as drivers jumped out of their cars to shout with joy.[8] But not long after, the hastily approved vaccine infected 220 children with polio, and public trust in clinical experimentation started to deflate.[9] Revelations of unethical trials followed—exposés of the government-sponsored Tuskegee Syphilis Study in the early 1970s proved a historical nadir—and disillusionment hardened into dislike. Today, although Americans buy on average more than ten prescriptions every year, less than one in twenty are willing to take part in the clinical trials that separate the dangerous drugs from the life-saving ones.[10]

Less than 4 percent of cancer patients, who generally have the most to gain from new experimental treatments, volunteer for experimental drug trials, a rate industry insiders deride as "appallingly low." Many people with cancer "simply didn't want to move from their homes to the clinical center for the time—sometimes weeks—necessary to participate in a trial," noted industry journal *Scrip*. Others, particularly elderly patients, felt that "cancer may be a sign they have lived long enough."[11] Even trials for what would turn out to be breakthrough cancer drugs like Genentech's breast-cancer drug Herceptin almost withered and died for lack of willing subjects. "Every year tens of millions of women die from breast cancer, and they couldn't get a hundred subjects for a trial," clinical research exec Dennis DeRosia recalls bitterly.[12]

The unmentioned reality is that cancer patients are hardly irrational in judging new drugs unworthy of their trouble. Despite the huge amount of investment in cancer research, "success has largely eluded us," admitted industry scientist David Horrobin. "The few outstanding successes in rare cancers cannot hide the overall failure."[13] For many other conditions, useful drugs are already in adequate abundance. Americans might be convinced to try a new brand-name drug after absorbing a vigorous marketing campaign touting it as the second coming, but when it is a lowly, unapproved experimental medicine, why should they bother? Most patients were uninterested in testing out Pfizer and Eyetech's new eye-disease drug Macugen, for example, because there were already many other drugs available and Macugen had to be injected directly into their eyes. Besides, there were at least two other trials for the same kind of drug, with different delivery systems, going on at the same time.[14] So scarce have willing subjects become in the West, Horrobin wrote in a 2003 *Lancet* paper, that some drug companies have taken to aggressively recruiting more subjects than they need, a preemptive strike against rivals on the hunt for warm bodies to fill their test clinics.[15]

Today, industry investigators can count on failing to find sufficient numbers of willing test subjects on time in four out of five of their clinical trials, and the financial strain of hunting for increasingly disinclined test subjects threatens to render the entire industry moribund. While the annual cost of drug development remains mired in controversy, undisputed is the fact that the price tag has zoomed steadily upward since at least 1980, while the output of new FDA-approved drugs has remained essentially stationary. And every day a new drug remains locked in development bleeds companies of up to $1 million in potential sales income.[16]

Western medicine has relied on human and animal experimentation since ancient times. It was by dissecting the bodies of criminals and the poor, for example, that Greek physicians discovered the nervous system in 300 B.C.[17] But it was only after the rigorous experimental design called the controlled clinical trial emerged in the 1940s and was codified into U.S. law in 1962 that the global hunt for experimental bodies began in earnest. After a brief period of testing experimental drugs on the U.S. prison population, a practice which ended when ethical scrutiny of trials was stepped up in the 1970s, most drug companies partnered with university hospitals and academic doctors to conduct trials. University doctors were the best experts to call on: reputed to be beyond reproach ethically, they had the patients at their fingertips, the know-how to design and conduct scientifically sound trials, and enough perceived independence to lend weight and credence to the findings.

But over the course of the 1980s and 1990s, the drug market skyrocketed. By 1989, for example, drug companies were angling to launch more than three times more drugs on the market than they had back in 1970. Impatient drugmakers started to get tired of their ponderous academic partners. "Pharmaceutical firms are frustrated with academic medical centers," University of California's Thomas Bodenheimer noted in an influential 2000 *New England Journal of Medicine* paper. "Slow review of industry proposals . . . delays the starting dates of trials." Academic hospitals "have a bad reputation," according to Greg Fromell, who works at a company specializing in running drug trials for the industry. They "overpromise and underdeliver."[18]

By the late 1990s, the flow of cash from drug companies to academic medical centers had slowed to a trickle, the stream diverted to a new breed of faster, more aggressive drug trial entrepreneurs. New outfits like Quintiles Transnational and Covance call themselves "contract research organizations" (CRO). For a fee they take a drug company's blueprints for a clinical trial and promptly deliver patients, investigators, and results in return.[19] "At Quintiles," the company's Web site says, "we know it's all about results. That's what you want. And that's what you'll get, on schedule or maybe even a little ahead of it." Some CROs even insert trial results into FDA applications and splice them into prestigious journal articles on behalf of their industry clients.[20]

At first, CROs performed this trick by capitalizing on a previously unexploited pool of potential subjects: the millions of patients treated at local clinics and private practices by community physicians. Then they slowly started to look beyond U.S. borders. After all, the FDA had long allowed drug companies to submit data from clinical trials conducted outside the United States, in 1987 even going so far as to accept a new drug application with data solely from overseas trials. Back then there had been no big stampede abroad, as academic investigators considered data from developing countries unreliable. Not so the new CROs.[21]

Just as automakers and apparel manufacturers had fled the stringent labor and environmental laws of the West to set up shop in the developing world, drug companies and CROs streamed across the border. Although companies aren't required to alert the FDA before testing their drugs on non-U.S. patients, nor does the FDA track research by location after approving new drugs, it is clear that the tectonic plates have shifted.[22] Between 1990 and 1999 the number of foreign investigators seeking FDA approvals increased sixteenfold, the Department of Health and Human Services' Office of the Inspector General found.[23] By 2004, the FDA estimated, drug companies angling for FDA approval of their new products were launching over sixteen hundred new trials overseas every year.[24] The most popular destinations are not Western Europe and Japan, but rather the broken, impoverished countries of Eastern Europe and Latin America.[25] Russia, India, South Africa, and other Asian and African countries have proven equally fruitful.

Between 2001 and 2003 the number of trials conducted in the United States—and the number of investigators hired to oversee them—plummeted. While U.S.-based investigators dropped by 11 percent, the number of investigators abroad fattened by 8 percent.[26]

By 2006, GlaxoSmithKline, Wyeth, and other drug giants predicted, half or more of their trials would be conducted overseas.[27]

Fleeing the empty test clinics of the West, drugmakers who have set up shop abroad wallow in an embarrassment of riches. The sick are abundant, and costs are low. In India, "apart from the low-cost of field trials," enthused a Pfizer press release, "a billion people means there is never a shortage of potential subjects."[28] In South Africa, a leading CRO noted on its Web site, patients suffered "an extremely high prevalence of HIV/AIDS and other major diseases including cardiovascular, diabetes, hypertension, mental illness and cancer." Their lack of access to medicines made them particularly appreciative of the free drugs offered in trials, no matter how experimental. "The vast majority of people have only the most basic healthcare," the Quintiles Web site noted, allowing "clinical trials [to] provide study participants with access to more sophisticated medicine."[29]

Many patients in developing countries don't balk at the discomfort of experimental procedures either. In the United States investigators reject protocols that require that their subjects undergo painful, invasive procedures. Bradley Logan, MD, who runs drug industry trials on contract, remembers being approached to conduct a trial that required that he surgically insert telescopic devices into women's abdomens that were ten times bigger than he and other doctors had been using for years. "I said no. I'm not making this big hole in a woman when it isn't necessary," he said, outraged.[30] "I've seen protocols that require five endoscopic biopsies in a single month," another industry researcher complained to CenterWatch. "Is it reasonable to assume that enough patients will willingly submit to this regimen to meet enrollment targets?"[31]

Not so elsewhere on the planet. "We did a study in Russia and the U.S.," said Wurzlemann. "But we got a lot more patients in Russia, because patients had to get a venogram," that is, tolerate the surgical insertion of an intravenous catheter that would administer contrast-heightening chemicals so investigators could better scrutinize their X-rays. In the United States venograms have been largely replaced by noninvasive CT scans and MRIs. "The Russian people were happy to do this, as other alternatives are not available," Wurzlemann proclaimed. Yuri Raifeld, Wurzlemann's Russian colleague, who was sitting in the audience, chortled. "Well, I would not say they were happy to do it," he said, "but they did it!"[32] The room tittered.

And so, in contrast to the agonizingly slow pace of enrollment in trials at home, recruitment abroad is rapid. In South Africa Quintiles herded 3,000 patients for an experimental vaccine study in just 9 days. They inducted 1,388 children for another trial in just 12 days.[33] And unlike American patients, who hemmed and hawed and often simply dropped out of studies, in India, boasted Vijai Kumar, head of a New Delhi–based industry trial center, "we have retained 99.5 percent of the subjects enrolled."[34]

In 2003, Pfizer announced plans to set up a global clinical trial hub in India.[35] GlaxoSmithKline and AstraZeneca followed suit, dispatching teams to set up new clinics and offices on the poverty-stricken subcontinent.[36] Glaxo aimed to relocate up to 30 percent of its gargantuan clinical trial business to "low-cost" countries such as India and Poland, its CEO said in 2004, saving the company over $200 million a year.[37]

On their heels followed an army of CROs, one-third of which set up shop in foreign countries between 2000 and 2002.[38] Headquartered in North Carolina, Quintiles littered new clinics and offices across the developing world in Chile, Mexico, Brazil, Bulgaria, Estonia, Romania, Croatia, Latvia, South Africa, India, Malaysia, the Philippines, and Thailand. Covance boasted that it could run trials in over a dozen countries at twenty-five thousand separate medical sites worldwide. New outfits like Neeman Medical International advertised its "access to large, previously untapped patient populations" in Latin America and Asia. "Ski where the snow is," a Neeman advertisement advised. "Conduct clinical trials where the patients are."[39]

Trade shows and conferences dedicate themselves to supporting the new trend, while the industry press regularly runs encouraging advice and how-to tips, from "Success with Trials in Poland" and "Organizing Large Randomized Trials in China: Opportunities and Challenges" to "Clinical Trials in Latin America: Meeting the Challenges Can Reduce Time-to-Market," "Discover Russia for Conducting Clinical Research," and "A billion-dollar clinical research opportunity lies in India."[40]

Developing countries, South African bioethicist Carel Ijsselmuiden says, have become "a great, global lab."[41]

Is there anything intrinsically wrong with drugmakers or other Western medical researchers taking advantage of the disparity between a drug-wealthy healthful West and a med-famished global poor if patients consent, none are harmed, and some may even be helped a little bit? Clinical researcher Malcolm Potts, PhD, thinks not. In a February 2000 paper Potts advocated stripping away health protections for subjects in developing countries in order to speed trial results to investigators. Part of his rationale hinged on a typical—and selective—fatalism. "The real world is exceedingly painful," he noted.[42] That is, the ill health of the developing world, which is now proving valuable for Western science to mine, is something mournful perhaps, but as static and irreversible as the setting sun. And yet, it is almost fully a product of a just a few centuries of political and economic machinations.

Just a few centuries ago Westerners were a fairly sickly bunch. Most could expect to live just twenty-five years. As medical historian Roy Porter explains in his classic 1997 tome, *The Greatest Benefit to Mankind: A Medical History of Humanity*, by unleashing the diseases of the old world upon the new, and introducing African pathogens from the bodies of their imported slaves, Western colonists vanquished as much as 90 percent of some of the native populations of the Americas. Slashing forests, capturing workers, and unleashing wars and streams of refugees in Asia and Africa, Western colonists spread and deepened local diseases such as kala-azar, bilharzia, cholera, and sleeping sickness. New medicinal plants and materials from the colonies were added to the Western pharmacopoeia. From Brazil came the emetic ipecacuanha; from Peruvian tree bark, the first-ever specifically effective medicine, malaria-curing quinine.[43]

Thus enriched, Western powers intensified their consumption of the planet's iron, wood, and coal, fashioning them into tools that would remake their rough-and-tumble medical practices, and revolutionize their health status. Early microscopes by the mid-1860s allowed French scientist Louis Pasteur to connect the ceaseless activity of microorganisms to the onset of disease, an insight that social crusaders put into action with widespread campaigns to separate the microbial pests from the humans they preyed upon. Before the 1900s most Europeans, living in squalor, drinking contaminated water, and being tended by bloody-handed doctors and surgeons, could hope to live no more than thirty years. One in five infants didn't survive birth. By the 1920s simple methods of avoiding pathogenic microbes—washing with soap and water, separating wastes from drinking water, throwing out spoiled foods—had extended most Western lives until well into their fifth decade.[44]

Such efforts languished in the colonies. In most colonies "the European administration attempted to separate from the prevailing environment," public health expert Oscar Gish writes, "ensuring sanitary conditions in their own living areas but very often creating a sanitary cordon between itself and the surrounding native quarters."[45] In India, for example, British administrators blamed the epidemics of cholera and malaria among the locals on Indians' "filthy habits," disregarding the fact that many had been forcibly resettled on mosquito-infested swamps.[46] The British had cleared marginal lands of forests and cut tens of thousands of miles of canals, which were devoid of drainage ditches, for the irrigated farmland and railroads that transformed India into a productive colony for the crown.[47]

World War II closed the age of empire. But Western health interventions—now sent under the rubric of aid—didn't always reverse the earlier trend. Disastrous malaria eradication campaigns such as the 1950s World Health Organization (WHO) effort, eloquently documented in journalist Laurie Garrett's book *The Coming Plague,* intensified rather than alleviated the burden of malaria in Asia. In 1961, at the height of the campaign, India suffered fewer than 100,000 cases of malaria; by 1977, after the doomed effort was abruptly canceled, the country's caseload topped 6 million.[48] The WHO's 1966 smallpox eradication program, while successfully ridding the world of that disease, involved forcible invasions of homes and the injection of live virus into fifty or more arms at a time.[49]

The current era of globalization has proven not much better. The World Bank and International Monetary Fund (IMF), with their billions of dollars in strings-attached loans, lay heavy hands on the health care of the global poor. According to the bank, "improved water and sanitation," the very public works that lifted the West out of its infectious soup, were "not particularly cost effective as a health measure."[50]

And so in Zaire, for example, World Bank and IMF "economic recovery" measures require the government to slash its spending on social services. In a single year the government fired more than eighty thousand teachers and clinicians. In Zambia, within just two years of such programs, the nutritional and health status of children had plummeted, canaries in a coal mine.[51] Infant mortality rose by 25 percent while life expectancy dropped from fifty-four to forty years.[52] In Argentina, polio and DPT immunizations fell by nearly 25 percent between 1992 and 1998, and throughout Latin America previously controlled diseases such as cholera and dengue fever re-emerged at epidemic levels.[53] The flow of patients into clinics and hospitals in Nigeria, Kenya, and Ghana slowed to a trickle, dropping by half within days of the imposition of new fees. "Before, everyone could get health care," one patient in a developing country noted. "Now everyone just prays to God that they don't get sick because everywhere they ask for money."[54]

As wages fall, the price of goods increase, and social services shrink. Many indebted countries have fallen into violence and disarray, amid which the pernicious virus that causes AIDS has silently spread. By the turn of the century Africa would be home to more AIDS victims than anywhere else in the world. By at the very least failing to reduce poverty and at worst exacerbating it, some health economists say, World Bank and IMF loans had poured oil on HIV's fire. As one AIDS policy adviser plaintively wondered, "given the increased needs in terms of health on the continent, largely due to the prevalence of AIDS, why didn't the World Bank make *increasing* health budgets a condition for their loans?"[55]

Just as health care systems are being dismantled, multinational tobacco, soft drink, and fast-food companies have rushed into the emerging markets of the developing world, eased by international trade agreements forged throughout the 1990s. Sales of cigarettes in developing countries have skyrocketed, with many of the cigarettes sent to the developing world loaded with more addictive tar and nicotine than the ones allowed at home.[56] Coca-Cola aimed to become the number one beverage on the planet, buying up water licenses in poor countries where they could sell their nutritionally valueless drink for less than the price of a glass of clean water.[57] McDonald's spread its inexpensive, fatty, high-calorie foods across the globe, with four of its five new restaurants opened daily outside the United States.[58]

When a torrent of fast-food, soda, and cigarettes splashes into stagnant waters of malnourishment and poverty, a whirlpool of disease starts to swirl. Malnourished mothers tend to bear babies predisposed to storing excess energy as fat. This is a useful adaptive advantage in communities where calories might be scarce, as it can better enable babies to survive nutritional deficits. But when such babies grow up to consume Western-style diets chock-full of fatty, sugary foods, that benefit turns into a deadly burden, leading them to gain disease-causing extra fat much more rapidly than they would have otherwise.[59]

And so, hot on the heels of the soda makers has followed an epidemic of diet and lifestyle–related heart disease, diabetes, lung disease, and asthma, jostling ominously with infectious diseases already tamed in the West. Today, four out of five people who die of these chronic, noncommunicable diseases perish in developing countries. More Indians and Chinese suffer cardiovascular disease than Americans, Japanese, and Europeans put together. "As for overweight and obesity, not only has the current prevalence already reached unprecedented levels, but the rate at which it is annually increasing in most developing regions is substantial," a World Health Organization report noted in 2003. For developing countries barely treading water amid the flood of malnutrition, HIV infection, malaria, and tuberculosis, "the public health implications of this phenomenon are staggering," the WHO noted, "and are already becoming apparent."[60]

By 2000, tobacco-related diseases were felling ten thousand people every day—the vast majority of them, over two-thirds, in the developing world.[61] Diabetes and coronary heart disease had become epidemic in India, home to the greatest concentration of sufferers of Type II diabetes in the world. Twelve percent of the population was suffering from the condition, four times more than had been in the 1970s, costing the Indian government somewhere around $2.2 billion a year.[62] Worse, while diabetes in rich countries is primarily a condition of the elderly, in developing countries the disease strikes those in the prime of life, aged forty-five to sixty-five, slashing their average life expectancy by ten to fifteen years. In some areas of Africa as many as one in five people have diabetes, and nearly twenty million Africans suffer from hypertension.

In the middle-income countries of Latin America, the Middle East, and North Africa obesity has become as common as it is in the United States. By 1998, the World Health Organization deemed obesity, with all of its attendant health risks, to be a worldwide epidemic.[63]

Access to cheap medicines to address these ills is scarce. Multi-national drug companies eager to access the growing markets of

countries such as Brazil and India have pressured these governments to crack down on cheap local producers of medicines that
undercut their sales. The problem was especially acute in India,
where 1970s-era patent laws once protected only how products
were made—not the products themselves. The rule had allowed
local drugmakers who could reverse-engineer drugs to manufacture knockoffs of the latest brand-name drugs at a fraction of the
cost. The biggest Indian drugmakers, such as Cipla and Ranbaxy,
reverse engineered some of the most important medicines of
modern times, slashing the cost of treating AIDS from $15,000 a
year on patented, brand-name drugs to just a few hundred dollars.
What's more, bypassing the turf wars of brand-name companies,
who would as readily add a competitor's drug to their own as
Coke would add some Pepsi to its six-pack, the Indian drugmakers
had combined several different HIV medicines into combination
pills that could be administered in simple, once-daily doses.

When nonprofit health organizations and activist groups across
the developing world started importing the cheap, Indian-made
generic drugs the Western drug giants who had patented the compounds unleashed a firestorm of protest. In 1998, thirty-nine
multinational drug companies sued the South African government
for allowing the cheap drugs into the country.[64] By 2005, India,
along with other developing countries roped into World Trade Organization (WTO) agreements, would be forced to strike down its
relaxed patent laws, instituting instead twenty-year patent protection for drugs and other products. The vibrant generic drug industry is now crippled.[65]

In the end, each of these encounters with the West, from colo-
nization to globalization, played a part in producing the ideal human tabula rasa for drug-industry trials: bodies that were sick,
untreated, suffering the same diseases as those in the major drug
markets, and more likely to die of them to boot.

In South Africa, Boehringer Ingelheim taps into such patients at
its Lung Institute, a modern, airy building surrounded by an expansive parking lot in downtown Cape Town. Inside, two-story-high

glass windows throw shafts of sunlight onto a stylish seating area that is replete with the latest fashion magazines. In the well-appointed examining rooms, labs, and surgeries discreetly tucked down sparkling hallways, a well-paid staff conducts hundreds of clinical trials on new drugs for drug companies, from the latest anti-aging creams to allergy drugs and respiratory medicines.

The subjects for the institute's trials do not, on the whole, reside in the city of Cape Town itself, with its impeccable roads and dramatic skylines. Instead, most live in the gigantic, isolated shantytowns that ring the city, places where untreated disease runs rampant. One such shanty sits just yards from the edge of the national highway that speeds professionals from the tony white suburbs to the city of Cape Town. Handmade shacks patched together from found pieces of tin and cardboard jauntily sport the logos of the fancy appliances they had once encased. Tiny dirt alleyways wind between the dark one-room shacks. The people live cheek by jowl, until recently part of the 80 percent of black South Africans who don't have running water, the 50 percent who don't have electricity, and the 16 percent who have no toilet. (Nearly every residence housing a white or Asian in the country has access to all three amenities.)[66]

In some townships like this one more than one in five residents are infected with HIV, in aggregate forming the largest army of HIV sufferers on the planet. Spanish pharmacist Marta Darder works at an AIDS clinic a few miles away from the Lung Institute. Toiling out of a battered office in the sprawling township of Khayelitsha, she might as well be on another planet. "That is the schizophrenia of this country. It is completely divided," she said. The sounds of traffic and blaring pop music waft in through the open windows. The floors under Darder's feet are sagging and covered with threadbare carpeting.[67]

South Africans would need every ounce of resources from their public health facilities to rise to the challenge of the exploding AIDS crisis, Darder said. But many decimated public health facilities are increasingly turning to lucrative offers from the omnipresent, deep-pocketed drug industry instead. The case of the University of Cape Town's Groote Schur Hospital is typical. Back in 1967, the world's first heart transplant was conducted in the hospital's *Brazil*-like warren of padlocked buildings.[68] The apartheid government showered the institution with largesse. Over the years the mighty hospital grew to enjoy a budget of 450 million rand (around $70 million in today's dollars), an expanse of 3,600 beds, and the labor of 10,400 staff.

All that changed after apartheid fell. In the rush to privatize the economy and open it up to multinational companies, the hospital was devastated, along with much of the country's public health system. The facilities were splintered. Academic doctors fled for private practice. The staff shrank by 60 percent.[69]

Robin M. Pelteret, MD, a bushy-eyebrowed white South African physician, was hired in the early 2000s to help save the fallen facility—and in particular its ability to continue cutting-edge medical research—from ruin. Grants for vaccination programs or AIDS hospice care might provide a stream of funds, but Pelteret and the people who hired him had other ideas. "We need entrepreneurial opportunities," he said firmly.

"Research grants are not the most reliable," he said. "This faculty doesn't focus on the pure science but on clinical medicine . . . and we have huge numbers of people which have a unique profile for third world countries." The fluorescent tubes lighting the halls outside his office flicker on waiting black patients. Asian and white clinicians stride purposefully by. Pelteret said that the industry funding will subsidize public health research and services at the hospital, although clinicians such as Darder toiling in the townships profess skepticism.

Pelteret ensures that patients who show up at Groote Schur's public hospital looking for treatment are channeled into industry trials, at the hospital and at places like the Lung Institute. In return for referring patients and conducting industry experiments on them, the Groote Schur Hospital earns over 150 million rand—over US$20 million—every year.[70]

2

The Placebo Control

There's nobody more influential in determining how drug companies conduct clinical trials than legendary clinical trials expert Robert Temple, MD, a grizzled, mustached man in his midsixties with a vaguely groovy 1970s hairstyle. Now director of medical policy at the FDA, Temple's thinking has held sway at the FDA—and the international medical research establishment that looks to the FDA as a model—for over thirty years. He's judged countless new drugs, designed trial protocols, and written federal rules about them. Savvy investigators pay careful heed to the kinds of experimental data that Temple blesses, and design their trials accordingly. As a regulator and an analyst he has "made his mark," writes Philip Hilts in his history of the FDA, *Protecting America's Health*, "not just in American medicine but worldwide."[1]

Temple reserves his most unwavering support for the placebo-controlled trial design; that is, experiments in which one drug is pitted against an inert substance. Most investigators seek to shield subjects from the hazards of their experimental inquiries, but developing new drugs has never been a risk-free endeavor. Clinical research often puts investigators, who are also physicians, between a rock and a hard place. As physicians, they're obligated to provide their patients with the best care they can; but, as scientists, they must randomly assign one experimental method or some alternative not to help the patient per se but just to see what will happen.

That's why the only ethically acceptable circumstances under which a clinical researcher can assign a sick person to a placebo (or some other possibly inferior treatment) is when they really

18

don't know whether an active intervention will work any better, a state of confusion described as "equipoise." If researchers know that one option is better than the other, they are ethically obligated to simply administer it: failing to do so puts subjects—who are also their patients—in harm's way.

Nevertheless, in the wake of even the most wondrous new drug lies a trail of failed ones, their dangers revealed only through the bodies of living beings. Overall, 40 percent of new drugs that have already passed several rounds of testing in the laboratory nevertheless afflict human subjects with toxic reactions in Phase 1 trials.[2] Nearly half of Phase 3 trials of new drugs fail, exposing subjects to drugs that turn out to be ineffective or dangerous.[3]

The placebo-control orthodoxy promulgated by Temple and others boosts the peril. For in placebo-controlled trials, even if the experimental drug is safe and effective, some ailing subjects will have had to tolerate no treatment whatsoever, and the consequences for them can be dire indeed. For this reason, it is a trial design that has been attacked as unethical time and time again.[4]

Throughout the periodic skirmishes with activists and ethicists, though, Temple's support has been steadfast. As he's expounded in interviews, published papers, and conferences, for Temple placebo-controlled trials render the clearest data on whether a drug works or not in less time than any other kind of experiment. "We have very strong feelings on placebo," Temple said, "when people [in the trial] won't be harmed."[5]

But as the example of the drug nitazoxanide suggests, the harm considered tolerable for experimental subjects varies, depending in part on where in the world the subjects live.

Most new drugs, despite the aspirations of drugmakers, are neither wonder drugs nor blockbusters, but compounds that fall into the cavernous gray area in between: drugs with mostly subtle, fairly nonspecific effects on human physiology. Nitazoxanide is one such drug.

Jean-François Rossignol, MD, PhD, a drug developer for Smith-Kline Beecham, synthesized nitazoxanide in 1993. The molecule appeared to have some effect against parasitic infections, and a hopeful Rossignol jumped ship to start his own drug company, Romark Laboratories.

The new company's mission was to somehow commercialize nitazoxanide, turning it into "the foundation for a profitable pharmaceutical company," as newspapers based in the company's home state of Florida noted. First, Rossignol and his partner, investment banker Marc Ayers, coaxed $3 million from investors upon founding the company. Then, on the basis of early studies showing the drug's activity against intestinal parasites, they quickly got the drug approved in Mexico, netting another $10 million to further develop the drug.[6]

To turn the drug into a true success, though, the vast American market would have to be breached. The most likely pest that nitazoxanide might take on was a parasite called *Cryptosporidium*. Small even by parasite standards, *Crypto* wasn't even spotted by scientists until the early 1900s. The parasite burrows into cells in the intestines, reproduces rapidly, and then sheds tiny, dormant cysts that depart through the intestines, floating in sewage and pipes until taken up by another creature. In the mid-1970s scientists recognized with alarm that *Crypto* could perform this feat in human intestines as well as in animals. While parasitic infections on the whole are rare in the United States, when there are outbreaks, either *Crypto* or *Giardia* is the culprit.

In most people *Crypto*'s residency in the gut provoked diarrhea for a week or two, after which it would rapidly depart, leaving the host otherwise unscathed, and functional water filtration systems generally screened out the cysts anyway.[7] But every now and again, when water systems failed, the parasite could wreak havoc. In 1993, severe flooding in Milwaukee triggered an outbreak that sickened over half the population, killing 100 of the weakest and most vulnerable. One of the most daunting attributes of the parasite was its defiant resistance to disinfectants: in fact, scientists prepared pure samples of the parasite by mixing *Crypto*-infected stool with undiluted bleach.[8]

But Romark wouldn't have to wait for periodic water department meltdowns to sell nitazoxanide for cryptosporidiosis. In immune-compromised AIDS patients crypto could be devastating. The parasite could settle in for months, even years. And the diarrhea it caused was explosive and uncontrollable. A bite of an unwashed fruit or an innocent nuzzle from a contaminated farm animal, and HIV-infected people would find themselves rushing to the toilet day and night, the great volumes of water exploding from their intestines leaving them withered and dehydrated nearly to death. So uncontrollable was the crypto-induced diarrhea that while Rossignol and Ayers scrambled for funds, wasted AIDS patients with crypto were turning up at clinics wearing diapers. If nitazoxanide might work for these patients, it could be a lifesaver.[9]

By the mid-1990s Rossignol's company had started to test the drug in AIDS patients with crypto. They administered the drug to eighteen AIDS patients with diarrhea in Mali; four cleared the parasite.[10] When word got out to American AIDS doctors struggling with their suffering patients, they started to clamor for supplies of the drug. The FDA allowed nitazoxanide's distribution under a "compassionate use" program, whereby experimental drugs can be administered legally to patients with life-threatening illnesses if no alternatives are available. The minuscule Mali study with its four-out-of-eighteen odds hardly anointed nitazoxanide a miracle cure, but at the time the tug of HIV into the dark abyss of AIDS appeared as relentless as the tide. Patients and clinicians seized anything that might help.

Now Romark had scores of patients around the country taking its experimental compound. By carefully tracking how they fared, they might be able to use the data to garner FDA approval, especially in conjunction with data from a study of the drug about to be launched by researchers at the esteemed National Institutes of Health.[11] The government docs planned to enroll sixty AIDS patients with cryptosporidiosis, randomly assign them to receive either nitazoxanide or a placebo, wait a few weeks, and then compare their outcomes.[12] With its requirement that some patients crippled with crypto accept sugar pills from their doctors for weeks on end, the trial protocol was "not too friendly to people with AIDS, unfortunately," remarked Bill Bahlman, a founding member of ACT UP New York who served on a community advisory board for AIDS trials,[13] but would be a surefire way of proving to the agency that the drug was effective and worthy of approval.

But the NIH didn't move fast enough. By the mid-1990s the notion of slamming HIV with multiple antiretroviral drugs had been born, miraculously beating back many of the opportunistic infections that debilitated and killed AIDS patients. Despite dramatic side effects, the difficulty of managing dozens of pills daily according to a strict schedule, and the $15,000 annual price tag for the drug cocktails, the mainstream press speculated that "this ordeal as a whole may be over," as social critic Andrew Sullivan wrote in the *New York Times Magazine*. Was it "the End of AIDS?" as *Newsweek* magazine asked on its cover?[14] Deep in the antipodes researchers wondered whether an onslaught of antiretrovirals might vanquish crypto, too. Between 1995 and 1996 nine HIV-infected men in Sydney, Australia, rushing to the toilet with explosive crypto diarrhea between three and ten times a day, were treated with multiple antiretroviral drugs. Every single one cleared the parasite. Most gained up to thirty pounds.[15]

And yet, despite the startling success of combination antiretroviral therapy, the NIH plodded onward with its placebo-controlled trial of nitazoxanide, trolling for *Crypto*-infected AIDS patients for the experiment in the spring of 1997. If the NIH trial had struck AIDS activists as unfriendly before, now it seemed downright repugnant. With the potent new therapy on offer, only the most altruistic or impoverished AIDS patients suffering with crypto would risk the chance of being given a placebo. By the spring of 1998, with only ten patients on board, the NIH was forced to abandon the trial.

Between Romark's founding in 1993 and May 1998, when the FDA advisory committee finally met to review data on nitazoxanide, everything had changed. Romark presented its data on nitazoxanide without any data from the aborted NIH trial. The committee was less than impressed. The drug hadn't cured any patients of cryptosporidiosis. The best that Romark had been able to prove was that the drug eased the diarrhea, lessening the number of trips to the toilet for a little over half of the patients who took it. Since the company had no data on how the patients who took the drug compared to others not given the drug, it was possible that even the weak salutary effect had nothing to do with the drug whatsoever, FDA advisers argued.

"We're interested in controlled comparisons," announced the FDA's statistician, Nancy Silliman; that is, data showing how the drug works in contrast to how another drug—or placebo—works. "The interpretation of uncontrolled data," such as Romark had presented, "is problematic at best," she said. The only way to be able to tell for sure whether nitazoxanide worked, she and other FDA advisers maintained, was with a placebo-controlled trial such as the NIH had planned—and which was scuttled due to lack of interest.[16]

Silliman's dismissive posture exasperated Rosemary Soave, MD, a cryptosporidiosis expert who had presented the data on nitazoxanide to the committee. Soave found the whole idea of a placebo-controlled trial for crypto in AIDS patients distasteful. "It was really very difficult to ask them to enroll in a trial where they would postpone getting a potentially effective agent for as long as perhaps three weeks," she said. "This is three weeks of suffering that most patients who are in this condition and have numbered days ahead of them are really not willing to do. . . . And that is really understandable." Placebo-controlled trials for such a dire condition, when evidence suggested that drug therapy could help, were "very difficult, if not impossible," she told the committee. "Many physicians and patients feel it is totally unethical."[17]

But the FDA committee wasn't interested in such dilemmas, Soave said. They "didn't pay one bit of attention when I was trying to explain how tough it was for the patients," she remembered later.[18] The committee rejected Romark's application. Perhaps the drug could be tested against placebo elsewhere, one committee member suggested. "I think consideration has to be given to the international setting," said Johns Hopkins gastroenterologist Cynthia Sears, "where HIV is rampant and additional therapies are obviously not available in many instances."[19]

Disappointed, Soave soon moved on. There wasn't much more work to be done on AIDS and cryptosporidiosis anymore anyway, she thought. With combination antiretroviral therapy the most effective way to cure opportunistic infection, she said, "a lot of these drugs went by the wayside."[20]

Romark took the blow in stride. They could still capture $100 million in sales every year if they could get the drug approved, Rossignol told reporters. All they had to do was find a new market. Crypto may have stopped being a serious problem for AIDS patients, but it was still a nuisance for the handfuls of Americans, particularly children, who caught the bug from dirty swimming pools, farm animals, or unwashed fruits. If delivered in a three-day course of sweet, strawberry-flavored syrup, nitazoxanide prescriptions might be eagerly snatched up by frustrated parents caring for intestinally challenged toddlers.

But running trials that might satisfy the FDA would be daunting in the United States. Cases of cryptosporidiosis had become rare, sporadic, and dispersed. Enrolling sufficient numbers of sickened patients would require the help of thousands of physicians across the country, each of whom might pass months if not years before seeing a single case. Romark didn't have hundreds of millions of dollars to spend on developing the drug, unlike the big pharmaceutical companies. They had $40 million.[21]

And so Romark's hunt for bodies began. It began in Romark's home state of Florida and ended in a small, impoverished country in sub-Saharan Africa.

When the British left Zambia in 1964, the country was "little more than a hole in the ground" where copper veins had been mined, a government official remembered. Infrastructure, save whatever was required to claw out the copper, was minimal.[22] The new government set about bringing the copper mines and farms back under Zambian control, building bridges and roads, and providing water services, free education, and free health care to a populace that would grow to ten million strong. Soon the country was one of the richest in all of sub-Saharan Africa,[23] boasting two universities, as well as a medical school and university teaching hospital located in the dusty capital city, Lusaka.[24]

But the country was dangerously dependent on income from selling copper, and when copper prices collapsed while the price of the petroleum products needed to run the mines spiked in the early 1970s, the country rapidly descended into debt. By 1980, Zambia's external debt had skyrocketed from $800 million in 1970 to over $3 billion, and desperate government officials turned to the IMF and World Bank for relief.[25] Over the following decades Zambia's nascent welfare state was methodically dismantled. More than 250 formerly government-run programs were sold to private investors. Farmers were cut off from government-supplied fertilizers and other subsidies. Formerly free public clinics and hospitals started to charge hefty fees, whittling the flow of patients into health care facilities by 60 percent. Tens of thousands of government workers were retrenched, as the country waited for foreign investors to sense their opportunity and invest in rebuilding Zambia.

The investors came, but squeezing a profit out of Zambia's aging copper mines and embryonic infrastructure proved trying. The new mine owners promptly closed the clinics and hospitals the government used to run for the mine workers and their families. Some, such as mining giant Anglo-American, simply cut their losses and fled. Inflation ran at 100 percent by the early 1990s. Abruptly put out of work and suddenly bereft of government support, whole towns and cities collapsed.[26] By 1998, 73 percent of all

Zambians were living in poverty, and half of the populace was unable to scrabble enough food to meet their minimum requirements.[27] According to UNICEF, over a fifth of all Zambians risked death by starvation.[28] The flow of water and electricity to the capital city slowed to a sporadic trickle, creating conditions for paroxysms of cholera.

HIV began to spread as well. By 2003, 15 percent of the population harbored the deadly bug, including 150,000 children. The number of years Zambians could expect to live plummeted from over five decades in 1990 to less than thirty-five years by 2001, leaving the country with one of the shortest life expectancies of any country in the world.[29] The combination antiretroviral therapy that had effectively stanched the AIDS epidemic in the West had yet to arrive. In 2003, at least two hundred thousand Zambians were sick enough with AIDS to require immediate therapy with antiretrovirals, but the government was able to treat only six hundred patients.[30] A 2002 survey showed that 66 percent of Zambians had never even heard of antiretroviral drugs, let alone had the means to pay for them.[31]

The country's main hospital, the University Teaching Hospital in Lusaka, was at the forefront of dealing with the AIDS crisis, tracking the epidemic, offering testing and counseling when few in southern Africa were.[32] But its facilities were near collapse. Water and telephone services were sporadic. Shortages of medicines and equipment were so severe the hospital was deemed "nonfunctional," as Canadian journalist and Africa correspondent Jonathan Manthorpe put it.[33]

Thirty children perished every day in the hospital's pediatric wards, where as many as five infants might be found sharing a single oxygen tank.[34] The UN's special envoy for AIDS in Africa, Stephen Lewis, who visited the wards, described what he saw to a group of activists in late 2004.

Every 10 minutes there is an anguished howl that sears the psyche and you turn around and there's a woman kneeling by a cot, four and five infant kids in the cot, a combination of AIDS and famine in that particular situation. And she's weeping, and the nurse comes in with a white sheet and covers up the infant babe and takes the child away.[35]

It was, according to Lewis, "a scene from hell."[36]

The AIDS and infectious diarrhea that were killing the children stemmed from three interlocked aspects of their poverty: the lack of adequate food, the lack of clean water, and the lack of access to antiretroviral medicines. Untreated water teeming with a host of pathogens, from *Shigella* and cholera to *E. coli*, easily overcame the immune systems of weakened, hungry children, the resulting diarrhea draining them of nutrients and predisposing them to yet more intestinal infections and more diarrhea. The rampage of untreated HIV further weakened children's ability to fight off the parasites. Worldwide the deadly diarrhea-malnutrition-diarrhea cycle took the lives of two million children every year.[37]

But where foreign investors saw financial risks, Western medical researchers, including those that Romark would later employ, saw opportunity. Epidemiologists, virologists, and gastroenterologists all flocked to the University Teaching Hospital to set up studies in the new disease hotbed. "If you are going to study the problem, you go where the problem is the worst, and Africa was it," explained University of Texas infectious disease specialist Herbert DuPont, MD, who first jetted down to Zambia in 1992.[38]

"I like to travel. I like foreign things. I like exotic things," DuPont told a *Houston Chronicle* reporter in 1993. As an epidemic intelligence officer for the Centers for Disease Control, DuPont had been involved in the global malaria eradication program. "I'd much rather go to a developing country than Europe. I think there's a little bit of a missionary zeal too. I would really like to help people," he said. And Zambia was special, DuPont explained. Unlike elsewhere in southern Africa in the early 1990s, Zambian officials were relatively "open to any suggestions to save their nation" from AIDS. DuPont had tried to set up some research in

Zimbabwe, he recalled, but "we were not allowed to discuss sero-prevalence [the proportion of the population infected with HIV] or use the word vaccine." In Zambia, by way of contrast, DuPont said, "Anything is fair game. This is a special thing about Zambians—and the fact that they can only say yes."[39]

DuPont was not the only Western specialist excited by the research opportunities in Zambia. Like DuPont, University of London gastroenterologist Paul S. Kelly had set up research collaborations with clinicians at University Teaching Hospital in Lusaka. It was Kelly whom Romark employed to run its trial on how nitazoxanide worked against crypto in children.[40] At Lusaka's University Teaching Hospital Romark found something special. The sad tide of sick children washing over the hospital, the company announced in a press release, comprised a "consistent and controlled study group" for their drug.[41]

Between November 2000 and July 2001 thousands of parents straggled into Lusaka's clinics and hospital, clutching tiny bundles: their shrunken, malnourished babies and toddlers whose innards, it seemed, were seeping out. Kelly and his Zambian colleagues screened them all, hoping to find a sufficient number who were infected with *Crypto*. Outside, the rutted roads overflowing with water had turned into orange swamps.[42] Of the over fifteen hundred children suffering from diarrhea who had staggered into the hospital and clinics, Kelly found one hundred who were willing to be part of his study.

The toddlers whose parents agreed to enroll them in the trial in Lusaka were extremely ill. They'd been plagued with diarrhea for days. Most were severely underweight. Half were infected with HIV. The children were dying.

Romark's studies of nitazoxanide in Egypt and Peru had shown the drug to be remarkably effective against *Crypto*, at least in non-HIV-infected patients. In Egypt, the drug had cured around 80 percent of the subjects;[43] all they seemed to need was a three-day course of the drug.

Treating the HIV-infected children with crypto in Lusaka would prove more challenging. Rosemary Soave's studies had shown some limited effectiveness when the drug was administered for weeks and even months at a time. Kelly's own investigations, one of which he'd published in 1996, had found that a two-week course of another drug, albendazole, helped alleviate the diarrhea in such patients, too.[44]

As per the study protocol, Kelly gave nitazoxanide to twenty-five of the children—those who were HIV free—for three days. Fourteen improved within a week. The other eleven children, given a second three-day course, likewise improved. The drug had, arguably, saved their lives.

Twenty-two other children, their bodies wasted with crypto, were not as lucky. These children had fallen into the placebo group. Besides the fluids and vitamins that all diarrhea patients got, these children were given nothing. A week later, four were dead.

The fate of the HIV-infected children in the trial was worse. Twenty-five were given a short, three-day course of the drug, despite evidence that suggested such a short course wouldn't work. Five perished. Another twenty-four of the HIV-infected children didn't even get the three-day course. They got placebos. Four died.[45]

It would be useful to know how the surviving children and the relatives of the dead felt about the experiment after it was all over. Did they know, as their doctors must have, about the evidence that better cures for their children could have been had with anti-retroviral therapy, lengthy treatment with nitazoxanide, or alternative drugs such as albendazole? Was the history of the drug and the experiment—the facts that patients in the United States had refused to be involved in an experiment such as this, and that it was designed to launch a drug aimed at societies far distant from their own—made clear to them? These are unknowns. Their experiences, save perhaps for a few lines of technical data, went unrecorded. Like so many experimental subjects in poor countries, they melted back into a social sphere that science rarely penetrates.

* * *

Two central tenets of medical research sealed the fates of the children enrolled in the nitazoxanide trial in Zambia. The first is that clinical trials should be randomized and controlled, a standard that doomed Romark's early, uncontrolled trials, and forced it to revamp its drug for a new market. The second, articulated most forcefully in recent years by Robert Temple among others, is what compelled the drugmaker and the investigators to leave U.S. shores in search of patients who wouldn't balk at being given inert compounds. It's a corollary of the first tenet: within randomized, controlled clinical trials, the very best thing to give to the control group, from a scientific point of view, is a placebo.

In a randomized controlled trial (RCT) subjects are randomly assigned to receive either the experimental drug or some other intervention. Both groups are treated exactly the same in all other respects save for this one difference. Then, whatever difference emerges in how the two groups fare can fairly be attributed to the experimental intervention.[46] To cancel out any bias researchers might have in assigning subjects to one or the other group, or might inadvertently impart to subjects while in the study, RCTs are often "double-blind," meaning that neither subjects nor clinicians know which subjects are receiving the experimental drug and which aren't. After the trial period lapses investigators "unblind" the study and see which group did better.[47]

Patients around the world can thank the RCT for convincing Western physicians to abandon the medicine by anecdote and received wisdom that reigned for millennia, during which blood letting, earthworms rolled in honey, owl brain, deer heart, fox lung, goat liver, powdered human skulls, rabbit testicles, cow dung, and the fresh blood of a dying Christian gladiator passed for medical treatment.[48] Only a precious handful of these enthusiastically prescribed regimens—salicin from willow bark, digitalis from foxgloves, quinine from cinchona bark—would later be proven to treat pain and disease effectively.[49]

That allopathic medicine works at all owes much to the RCT. The experimental design, which first emerged in London in 1946, is "nothing less than the single most important development in the revolution of modern therapeutics," wrote Harvard pharmacologist Jerry Avorn—"the most powerful intellectual medicine we have."[50]

It is possible to conduct RCTs successfully by providing an alternative treatment for subjects in control groups, but according to Temple and Kelly, using placebos as a control renders the most unequivocal data. And yet, deciding what to use as a control has not always been driven primarily by scientific considerations. Politics often grabs front seat.

Take, for example, the 1954 trials of Jonas Salk's experimental polio vaccine, the RCT's big national debut. Polio wasn't a huge killer at the time, but as a crippler of the young, particularly those of the upper and middle classes, it was a terror-inducing scourge, forcing communities to shut down their swimming pools and movie theaters at the height of the summer's polio season. Salk's sponsor, the March of Dimes, aware that leading virologists were skeptical of the experimental vaccine—it consisted of the entire, virulent polio virus itself rather than a similar virus that could train the body to fend off more dangerous foes—was eager to produce the most convincing data possible.[51] A double-blind RCT would be ideal, a "beautiful . . . experiment over which the epidemiologist could become quite ecstatic," as Salk put it.[52] The plan was to give the control group placebos. Nobody really knew if Salk's vaccine worked anyway, so it wasn't as if they'd be depriving anyone of some known effective medicine. For all they knew the vaccine might even hurt the children: those randomized to placebo might have better outcomes than those in the vaccine group.

But just as Romark and the NIH discovered years later when they attempted to run a placebo trial for nitazoxanide among U.S. AIDS patients, the majority of the state health departments approached about running the trial in their public school systems objected to the placebo control. So great was their faith in Salk and the March of Dimes that they wanted *all* of their enrolled children to get the vaccine, experimental or not.[53]

Salk, publicly at least, agreed with the underlying sentiment: denying the experimental vaccine to any child would be a travesty, indeed. The placebo-controlled design, he said, "would make the humanitarian shudder," he opined.[54] The compromise the foundation settled on was less rigorous but more politically palatable, involving an awkward mix of two concurrent trials: a large-scale trial in which all participants would be vaccinated, and a smaller one that compared vaccinated children to those injected with placebos.[55]

The same year, Louis Lasagna, MD, called by some the father of modern pharmacology, discovered the "placebo effect," the phenomenon by which patients are healed by inert compounds, and became a forceful advocate for more rigorous standards for drug approvals. For Lasagna, as for Temple later, trials that pitted an experimental drug against an alternative treatment too often told scientists nothing. "In the absence of placebo controls, one does not know if the 'inferior' new medicine has any efficacy at all," Lasagna wrote in a 1979 editorial. " 'Equivalent' performance may reflect simply a patient population that cannot distinguish between two active treatments that differ considerably from each other, or between active drug and placebo." In his myriad appearances at congressional hearings, Lasagna urged the FDA to require placebo-controlled trials for all new drugs.[56]

Today, the FDA's position is that it prefers placebo-controlled trials, if they are ethical and feasible.[57] Temple took the baton as placebo-control advocate from Lasagna, who died in 2003. And now, the placebo-control orthodoxy is firmly entrenched, with a number of novel arguments forwarded in its favor. Kelly, for example, was certain that using placebos in Lusaka was the right thing to do. "There is no other way of being absolutely sure that the stuff actually works," he says. "It is very very important to do this in third world countries, for two reasons. One, because if you misguide people into thinking that your drug works when it doesn't, you'll be responsible for diverting precious resources away from something else which may also be important. Two, we cannot assume that something which works in other countries will work here. . . . There are geographical differences and we have to be sure that it works where we're planning to use it."[58]

There are other rationales that are somewhat less lofty. Most new drugs are not miraculous cures like penicillin, or a shot of insulin to a comatose diabetic. For most, the margin of effectiveness is narrow, colored in shades of gray. "I'm not used to finding black and white," agrees Rosemary Soave. "You usually have to struggle to find the difference" between patients who got the drug and those who didn't.[59] Anecdotal evidence might be sufficient in the case of a wonder drug, but discerning how a weakly acting drug works requires the precision, and relatively low expectations, of a placebo-controlled trial.

For drugmakers, the choice is obvious. "Why risk trying to be better than something," an FDA medical officer noted, "when all you need to show is that you are better than nothing?" Sure, patients randomly selected to get placebo rather than an active drug might suffer a bit—in trials for new diabetes drugs, for example, investigators withheld active drugs from their subjects in order to worsen their hyperglycemia before testing a new drug on them— but "in the absence of permanent harm, why should a federal agency restrict the right of a patient to participate in a clinical trial?"[60] So long as the patients are adequately informed that they might get a placebo, Temple insists, there is nothing ethically troublesome about a placebo-controlled trial. "I think it is usually good for people to be in clinical trials," Temple says optimistically.

Romark brought its results from the nitazoxanide trial in Zambia, along with data from its trials in Egypt and Peru, to the FDA in May 2002, hoping to prove to the agency that the drug was worthy of approval. The regulators agreed. The drug, now dubbed Alinia, was launched in the United States in December of that year as a treatment for children infected with *Cryptosporidium* and another parasite called *Giardia*. For those children splashing in pools alongside toddlers wearing leaky diapers and the parents who had to look after them the short, three-day course of treatment would mean "less discomfort and less time away from work, school, and other activities," Romark's Web site announced. The company expected sales of $20 million in the first year, $50 million the following year, and sometime in the not-so-distant future, $100 million a year.

Alinia's value for children suffering from infectious diarrhea in Zambia and other developing countries is less clear. For scientists at the forefront of researching drugs and vaccines to treat infectious diarrhea in developing countries, such as those at the nonprofit Institute for OneWorld Health in San Francisco, nitazoxanide is an irrelevancy.[61] That's because, in most developing countries *Crypto* causes only about 5 percent of diarrhea cases in children under five years old, according to Johns Hopkins pediatric infectious diseases specialist Robert Black, MD. "And these are not particularly severe cases of diarrhea," he says.[62] Many of those who are harboring *Crypto* or *Giardia* are infected with a host of other intestinal parasites as well. A significant proportion is also infected with HIV. A drug whose effective use requires not only that patients harbor only one parasite but that clinicians actually know which one it is would understandably be of questionable value in places with limited diagnostic capabilities. In India, for example, where a vigorous local drug industry quickly made the drug available, the med is "nearly useless," says medical analyst Chandra Gulhati, MD.[63] Not to mention the fact that, according to independent researchers in Mexico, nitazoxanide had worse side effects with no greater efficacy than cheaper, older medicines.[64]

And yet it is true that unlike the scores of drugmakers seeking to muscle in to drug markets aimed at the aging rich of the developed world, Romark had developed a drug for a rare, parasitic disease, however imperfect. Few drug companies spent any time or money making drugs to neutralize parasites, aid workers struggling with onslaughts of parasitic diseases in tropical countries complain. But if Romark's hunt for experimental bodies had ended in Zambia, their market clearly began elsewhere. The children of Zambia shouldered the burden for nitazoxanide's development, but they are hardly beneficiaries of the drug's advantages, however fleeting. In Zambia, save for at the University Teaching Hospital, clinicians don't even bother trying to diagnose cryptosporidiosis in children with diarrhea. Nitazoxanide is not licensed for use in the country. Five years after the hospital had run the trial for Romark, they still had no supply of the drug.[65]

3
Growing the Pharma Monolith

Jill Weschler is a gray-haired, slightly hunched woman with a jokey manner. As an editor at *Pharmaceutical Executive* magazine she's well aware of the clinical research industry's reputation. Bioethicists think CROs are the "incarnation of evil," she says conspiratorially, in a nasal voice. "I mean, the gang at the *New England Journal of Medicine* think *no* trial should be done unless [health activist] Sid Wolfe does it!" She laughs. "I mean, who is clean enough?"

Weschler's point echoed a consensus that quickly emerged among the CRO investigators and executives chatting informally after Wurzlemann's talk in Washington, DC. The bad reputation is unfair, because subjects in industry trials are lucky. If patients are poor and medicine deprived, running a drug experiment on them is positively an act of charity. Isn't it more ethical, one demanded, "if patients are not getting any treatment that they are in clinical trials, if this is the only way they can get treatment?" "I was criticized for doing a *Shigella* trial," a former researcher for Schering commiserated. *Shigella* is a diarrhea-inducing bacterium that kills one million people around the world every year.[1] "They said you are taking advantage! But without that trial, those children would be dead!"[2]

The notion that clinical trials are not a burden for subjects but rather a fortunate opportunity to access new drugs pervades the clinical research industry. It stems, in part, from an underlying faith in the system of drug development to reliably churn out new drugs that are safe, effective, and useful. And yet, our patchwork regulations do little to ensure that this is the case. Rather than shaping the industry to reliably produce socially beneficial medicines, regulations have generally been applied in fits and bursts in the wake of drug-induced disasters. The industry has never been reined in coherently by law or incentive to produce the medicines we most need, at prices we can afford, and in recent years, many of our most stringent regulations and oversight mechanisms ensuring safety and efficacy have deteriorated in the shadow of an ever-growing pharma monolith.

That isn't to say that all new drugs are dangerous and ineffective. But it may not be feasible to rely on the drug-development system to ensure that the benefits of experimentation outweigh the risks. What's more, trends in the industry suggest that the margin of benefit for new drugs is rapidly shrinking, while the risks of experimentation remain constant or are even growing. And when there is a gap between risks and benefits, the global poor who are the subjects of today's body hunt pay the price.

Today, even though they aren't regulated as such, pharmaceutical products are valued in Western society as life-saving necessities like electricity and clean water, underpinning its unspoken toleration of the industry's growing hunt for bodies. That wasn't always the case.

For much of their first century of existence, drug companies were considered vaguely contemptible snake-oil peddlers. It was a fair enough assessment. Since opening their doors in the mid to late 1800s, drugmakers like Eli Lilly and Merck flogged mysterious "secret formulas," their actions and ingredients known only by catchy slogans and advertising jingles.[3] According to an 1885 survey, the main ingredients in these medicines were quinine and morphine. Merck sold cocaine; Bayer sold heroin.[4] Alcohol diluted with water was sold as a cure for colds, congestion, and tuberculosis. Only after these unregulated medicines had killed thousands of Americans, including countless infants who were given opiates, did Congress pass the 1906 Food and Drug Act, requiring drugmakers to list ingredients on their product labels.[5]

True "magic bullet" drugs, medicines that were selectively toxic rather than just diluted poisons, didn't emerge until 1932.[6] Sulfanilamide, a compound found in red textile dye, was the first compound that prevented bacterial cells from multiplying, allowing the host's immune system to destroy them. Laying waste to streptococcus, pneumonia, meningitis, and gonorrhea, sulfanilamide was dubbed by the *New York Times* "the drug which has astounded the medical profession."[7]

When one hundred children died from a sulfa concoction—Massengill had dissolved the drug in a sweet but poisonous solvent—Congress passed the Food, Drug, and Cosmetic Act of 1938, requiring toxicity tests for new drugs.[8] Not long afterward sulfa drugs were rendered ineffective by resistant strains of bacteria, and were replaced by penicillin, a drug with profound bacteria-killing properties. Penicillin's debut marked what Hilts aptly dubbed "the beginning of the faith."[9] Tuberculosis, already on the decline, was decimated. Syphilis, it appeared, might be stamped out as well. So effective was the drug against syphilis that the city of New York distributed the drug for free in its venereal diseases clinics starting in 1943. Within less than a decade the rate of syphilis infection in the United States had been quartered.[10]

Penicillin and the more potent antibiotics that followed it elevated public perception of drugmakers' products from snake oils to social goods.[11] Emboldened and now beloved, medical research—and the drug industry that relied upon it—stepped out of the shadows to become society's darling. The budget of the National Institutes of Health swelled from $180,000 in 1945[12] to $874 million by 1970.[13] NIH research provided new ideas and approaches for drug companies, and the resulting breakthroughs in industry labs garnered drug company scientists the Nobel Prize in medicine in both 1950 and 1952.[14] There appeared to be no disease that drug companies in partnership with medical science could not surmount, if nourished with enough time and funding.[15]

When it came to pricing, the drugs that emerged from this frenzy of medical research were not considered ordinary commodities.

New laws banned the advertisement of drug prices and reserved control over the use of the most potent drugs to physicians, rather than the patients and their insurers who would be handed the bill. Thus liberated from the yoke of sticker shock, all concerned consumed the novel meds—the new American birthright—in ever greater quantities.

By 1957, the drug industry was the most profitable industry in the country, with profit margins double the national average: 19 percent of investment after taxes. Drug sales "were unlike anything seen in the history of sales," wrote Hilts.[16]

The thalidomide disaster marked a turning point for the growing drug industry. While the scandal certainly revealed the folly of relying on lightly regulated, profit-seeking drug companies to protect public health, the legislation it sparked didn't require the industry to re-orient itself toward society's good health. Instead, the new rules required the industry to vastly step up the experimental activities held in such high esteem. Now the hunt for experimental bodies would begin in earnest.

The German company Chemie Grunenthal first started selling the sedative thalidomide under the trade name Contergan in 1957, claiming it was as powerful as a barbiturate but with no noticeable side effects.[17] In Europe and Africa Grunenthal promoted Contergan as being "as safe as mother's milk."[18] Thousands acquired the drug over the counter. Soon a small company called Vick Chemical and its subsidiary Richardson-Merrell decided to market the drug to pregnant women as a nausea treatment. The regulatory hurdles were not particularly taxing. No drugmaker had to prove in any way that their drug actually *worked*.

Richardson-Merrell started testing the drug's toxicity in animals. The results could not have been comforting: six of the eleven mice died; twenty-two out of thirty rats died; the dog died.[19] Reports also started trickling in from Europe that thalidomide was poisoning patients' nerves, resulting in tingling, numbed limbs, suggesting that the drug was penetrating the blood-brain barrier and could likewise cross into the placenta in pregnant women.[20] Nevertheless, the company launched a major clinical trial in early 1960, shipping the drug to over one thousand American doctors to administer to about twenty thousand of their patients. The company arranged for an obstetrician to sign off on a paper they had written about the drug, which would be published in the medical literature. The FDA, not convinced that the drug was truly safe, held up Richardson-Merrell's application, but American docs involved in the clinical trial continued to receive their thalidomide samples in the mail.[21]

Meanwhile, doctors outside the United States had grown increasingly alarmed at the rash of babies born with a once rare condition called phocomelia, in which hands and feet sprout directly from the body, like seal flippers. Many of the babies had no openings for ears, deformed intestines, and no bowel openings.[22] In 1961, an Australian obstetrician connected the outbreak to the use of thalidomide. It turned out that if taken even in a single dose during the first trimester of pregnancy, thalidomide could radically deform fetuses. The German news media splashed the story on its front pages.[23]

The American press didn't pick up the story until eight months later. By then, about forty babies had been born with phocomelia in the United States, including a handful under the care of the obstetrician who had signed off on the pro-thalidomide company medical paper. The FDA sent out investigators to recall thalidomide doses from doctors' offices, but the recall was a disaster. Most of the doctors hadn't even kept records of how much thalidomide they had received or doled out, and few managed to track down the doses from their patients.

Now lawmakers were forced to act. The bungled recall swept through a bill on drugs regulation, heralded by President Kennedy for allowing "the immediate removal from the market of a new drug where there is an immediate hazard to public health."[24] But the 1962 amendments to the Food and Drug Act required much more than quicker recalls of dangerous drugs. New drugs would not only have to prove themselves safe before being allowed on the market, they'd have to prove themselves effective as well. Anecdotal evidence or expert opinion wouldn't be sufficient either, but only randomized controlled trials in humans that proved a drug statistically better than a placebo. Companies would have to test their experimental drugs on animals first, then inform the FDA and secure consent from patients before embarking on human trials. Drugs approved between 1938 and 1962 would have to submit evidence retroactively showing that they worked or risk being forcibly banned from the market.[25]

The 1962 laws greatly enlarged the scale and number of experiments on humans, entrenching the randomized controlled trial as the basis for clinical experimentation. Safety studies could be adequately accomplished in a short time with just a handful of healthy volunteers. Now drug companies would have to convince sick patients to try experimental drugs, enroll them in massive trials, and give many of them placebos for comparative data. If the drug was aimed at some slowly progressing condition—heart disease, for example—data regarding its effectiveness wouldn't emerge for years. If the drug had but a small salubrious effect, documenting that it worked would require the participation of thousands, even tens of thousands, of patients. In 1938, companies wanting to prove to the FDA that their new drugs were safe could do so with slim applications that numbered just thirty pages. By 1968, companies that wanted to prove that their new drugs were both safe and effective would have to submit over seventy-two thousand pages of data to do it.[26]

While the new rules would do much to restore public confidence in the drug industry, ironically, the regulations did little to address the conditions that had led to the thalidomide disaster. Forty years later drugs that cause birth defects continue to slip past FDA regulators onto the market. Clinical trials rarely reveal such effects, since most trials exclude pregnant women, particularly when drugmakers suspect there might be a risk of birth defects. "The unfortunate reality is that we learn about virtually all teratogenic [birth defect–causing] effects only after a drug has already received marketing approval," Boston University epidemiologist Allen A. Mitchell wrote in the *New England Journal of Medicine* in 2003, "and of course only after it has been used by pregnant women."[27] A postmarketing surveillance system, Mitchell wrote, one which would have systematically caught early reports of nerve damage, is probably all that could have mitigated the disaster.[28]

Interest groups predictably complained that the new regulations were too strict. The American Medical Association argued that doctors, not impersonal trial results, should decide which drugs worked for their patients. Drug companies complained that the strict regulation would thwart their research efforts, as scientists would flee from industry labs. Undeterred, the National Research Council, tasked with evaluating the mountain of already approved drugs, ended up pulling no fewer than three hundred drugs. It wasn't just for a lack of evidence of efficacy, either: in some cases, companies had tested their drugs, found them to be ineffective, and marketed them anyway. Upjohn, for instance, marketed a combination of the antibiotic tetracycline and novobiocin, even though the company's own trials had shown that novobiocin counteracted the effectiveness of tetracycline.[29]

American faith in the promise of medical research proceeded with renewed vigor after the 1962 amendments, with the emergence of genetic engineering techniques—the cutting and splicing of strands of DNA—in the early 1970s.[30]

The biotech revolution soon ratcheted up the pace of drug development, enlisting the best minds of academia to do it. In 1978, Herbert Boyer, at the University of San Francisco, isolated the genes that instructed human cells to make insulin, synthesized them, and spliced them into bacteria, which started to churn out human insulin. Boyer didn't just write up a few papers and rest on his laurels. He and a colleague patented their discoveries and netted over $27 million in royalties.[31] With money from a savvy venture capitalist, Boyer founded a company to commercialize the technology. The company, Genentech, released "recombinant" insulin just four years later, in 1982, laying a foundation that would eventually make it one of the most successful biotech drug companies in the world.[32]

Before Boyer, academic researchers considered the commercial development of their research peripheral to their own careers. Back in the 1930s associations of the most esteemed scientists in pharmacology would refuse membership to anyone who even worked for a drug company.[33] Since Boyer, academic scientists have been patenting their discoveries, keeping them secret from colleagues, and starting up biotech companies to produce and market their drugs. In 1980, Congress pushed along the commercialization of academic research with the Bayh-Dole Act, aimed at promoting "collaboration between commercial concerns and nonprofit organizations." The new law allowed—and even obligated—universities to commercialize findings they made under the largesse of government grants by patenting them. Somehow, the thinking went, all of this activity would lead to major medical breakthroughs, such as a cure for cancer.[34]

Indeed, the flow of new drugs from the industry skyrocketed. Drugmakers deluged the FDA with more than twelve thousand applications to sell new drugs in 1989, compared to just forty-two hundred in 1970.[35] Between 1975 and 1985 more than eighty of the industry's new FDA-approved products and processes flowed from publicly funded academic research.[36] Prescription drug sales during those years tripled. The scale and pace of human experimentation to support the new drugs quickened in its wake.[37]

FDA rules facilitated the tsunami of new drugs flooding the market. In 1984, Congress passed legislation granting drug companies an additional five years of patent protection, balancing it with streamlined FDA review of generic drugs, which were meant to become quickly available after the lengthy brand-name patents expired.[38] But there were loopholes, which brand-name drugmakers exploited handily: the maker of a patented drug could sue any generic company seeking to produce the drug for patent infringement, automatically triggering a thirty-month stay on the production of generic meds.[39]

With guaranteed market monopolies secured, drug companies could invest more into selling big drugs for megamarkets. The only trouble was, while millions were dying from malaria, AIDS, and tuberculosis, those who spent the most on prescription drugs—aging Americans—were becoming healthier and healthier. Between 1965 and 1996 death rates from blocked arteries in the United States had dropped by 74 percent. Deaths from heart disease had dropped by 62 percent. Deaths from hypertension had dropped by 21 percent.[40]

How could drugmakers continue growing? If they did what the public had come to love them for—vanquishing sickness with curative wonder drugs—they'd have to make do with markets with minimal buying power, from the tuberculosis-ridden inner cities of the United States to malarial sub-Saharan Africa and tropical Asia. A more lucrative approach, albeit a smaller contribution to public health, would be to encourage wealthier, healthier customers to pop pills despite their relative vigor. After all, no FDA regulation requires drugmakers to invent high-priority drugs. As long as drug companies could prove their drugs safe enough and better than nothing in placebo-controlled trials, they could sell whatever kind of medicine they wanted, whether patients needed the drugs or not.[41] As the old pharma saying went, "While it's good to have a pill that cures the disease, it's better to have a pill you have to take every day."[42]

The industry slowly reoriented itself. The complaints and vanities of aging baby boomers and those over the age of sixty-five, who spent nearly three times more on pills, doctors, and hospitals than their younger cohorts, would call the shots, whatever drugs that could be marketed to them cashing in big.[43] With the right promotion, the new blockbuster drugs could bring in annual sales topping $1 billion each. Accordingly, the first modern blockbusters were not miracle cures like penicillin; they were the heartburn drugs Tagamet and Zantac.[44]

In 1985, a long-running government study on cardiovascular risk—the Framingham Heart Study—reported a correlation between low cholesterol levels and increased longevity.[45] It was just a correlation, of course, but the timing was perfect. Could it be that high cholesterol cuts lives short? Many Americans had high cholesterol levels, after all, and would likely maintain them given their penchant for fatty foods and sedentary lifestyles. If they could be convinced to take an expensive prescription drug every day for the rest of their lives—despite not feeling at all ill—Merck had just the drug for them.

First, the company planned what the *Washington Post* called "an advertising and public relations blitz" to paint cholesterol as Americans' top health adversary.[46] Then, in 1987, the company released Mevacor, a molecule called lovastatin that blocks an enzyme the body needs to make cholesterol. "It's going to be earthshaking," a cardiologist quoted by the *Wall Street Journal* enthused.[47]

It was. In its first year out, Mevacor brought in $175 million; by 1989, annual sales stood at $500 million. By 1991, Mevacor sales had topped $1 billion a year.

Besides showcasing how unhinged drug development was from promoting public health (better diets and more exercise would have conferred broader health benefits and was cheaper and safer to boot), Mevacor was a stunning testament to the power of marketing. For even while Mevacor sales spiked, experts continued to debate the pros and cons of high cholesterol levels. Some studies showed that people with high cholesterol actually lived longer than those with low cholesterol.[48]

Merck's trailblazing act of market expansion was soon followed by Eli Lilly's antidepressant Prozac, and a host of "lifestyle" drugs. These were drugs whose main medical innovation was their ability to be prescribed to millions, whether they were ill or not, or which accommodated rather than corrected for unhealthy lifestyles.[49] During the 1990s, Americans clamored for the new drugs, and showered the drug industry with its approval. *Fortune* magazine anointed Merck "the most admired company in America" every year between 1987 and 1993.[50] Amid the love fest, industry lobbyists, conservative economists, and patient advocates stepped up their criticisms of drugmakers' sole nemesis: the FDA. What would happen next would dilute the two most stringent standards for new drugs: that they prove themselves both safe and effective.

First the rules requiring proofs of efficacy were weakened. In a 1991 paper officials from the FDA's Center for Drug Evaluation and Research announced that new drugs would no longer have to prove that they alleviated disease and improved patient's lives. Now FDA regulators would be willing to allow drug companies to prove their drugs "worked" by showing that they possessed some quality more easily measured than the ability to make patients better, using what was called a "surrogate end point." Instead of having to prove that a new cardiovascular drug reduced mortality from heart disease, for instance, drug companies could show simply that the drug reduced cholesterol levels. Rather than show a new anticancer drug or AIDS drug extended patients' lives, they could prove instead that the drug shrank tumors or increased white blood cell levels.[51] Forget about time-consuming, patient-intensive trials on how drugs might work to help real patients in their struggle with illness: "The assessment of a new drug should flexibly evaluate safety and efficacy," the regulators wrote.[52]

With millions in pent-up sales hanging in the balance for every day a potential blockbuster drug was held up in trials, the FDA's new flexibility would prove highly lucrative for drug companies, although of questionable utility to patients. "There has recently been great interest in using surrogate end points . . . to reduce the cost and duration of clinical trials," wrote biostatisticians Thomas R. Fleming and David L. DeMets in a 1996 *Annals of Internal Medicine* paper titled "Surrogate End Points in Clinical Trials: Are We Being Misled?" "In theory, for a surrogate end point to be an effective substitute for the clinical outcome, effects of the intervention on the surrogate must reliably predict the overall effect on the clinical outcome. In practice, this requirement frequently fails."[53]

During the 1980s the FDA had approved two drugs to ease irregular heartbeats—Bristol-Myers Squibb's Enkaid and 3M's Tambocor—not because irregular heartbeats were considered dangerous in and of themselves, but because they were thought to lead to fatal heart attacks. Like shadows on a wall, irregular heart beats were surrogate markers for the fatal heart attacks. In 1989, after over two hundred thousand patients had been prescribed the drugs, an NIH-sponsored study found that no such linkage existed: not only did the drugs fail to extend patients' lives, they appeared to kill three times more patients than those administered placebos.[54]

Since then, numerous studies have exposed the hollow center of surrogate markers: drugs that lower cholesterol can increase mortality; drugs that reduce blood pressure increase patients' risk of heart attacks; AIDS drugs that increase CD4 counts have no effect on the course of the disease; and drugs that reduce tumors don't extend lives. And yet drugs that have proven they can do little more than alter these ghostly proxies continue to be approved by the FDA.[55]

Then, in 1992, with the passage of the Prescription Drug User's Fee Act FDA reviewers who painstakingly analyzed data on new drugs to ensure their safety were burdened with punishing deadlines. Under the new law drug companies would pay the FDA directly—up to $672,000 for each new drug application in 2005—in exchange for speedier deliberation times.[56] Regardless of the complexity of the drug or its safety profile, the FDA would be bound to meet strict new deadlines, shaving off weeks from review times and making the agency feel, as some insiders said, like a sweatshop.[57] Over the following years the average FDA review period for new drugs tumbled from thirty months to under seventeen, a neat deal for drug companies that could now count on many hundreds of millions of dollars in sales in exchange for the relatively paltry user fee.[58]

The rapid review times allowed dangerous drugs to slip through the FDA's fingers, critics complained, with increasing numbers of new drugs found to be life threatening only after they had been ingested by millions. In 1997, the FDA was forced to withdraw two drugs from the market after they injured and killed patients; in 1998, three drugs were withdrawn; in 1999, two were withdrawn; in 2000, no fewer than four drugs were withdrawn.[59]

The marketplace might have ably punished any drug company that produced meds that were marginally useful or unsafe with lackluster sales. But in 1997 came another regulatory change that circumvented such a correction.

Until 1997, the largest audiences for advertising messages—television viewers—were virtually unreachable for drugmakers. The FDA required that drug ads list, in addition to the therapeutic properties of the drug, all of its concomitant side effects. In a magazine ad, the side-effects list could be dispensed with effectively in the small type along the margins. In a television commercial, though, the list would have to be read out loud in excruciating detail. Few companies would attempt such a feat.

When companies tried, such as Hoescht Marion Roussel, they failed badly. In the early 1990s the company's best-selling prescription allergy drug, the nonsedating antihistamine Seldane, had been criticized for its dangerous side effects when taken in conjunction with other drugs. The FDA had decided not to pull Seldane off the market, despite its dangers, but things were looking bad for Seldane when, in 1993, Schering-Plough released a similar nonsedating antihistamine, Claritin, which quickly started to pull ahead in sales.

By 1996, Hoescht had a new product to take Seldane's place and counter the Claritin onslaught: the "new and improved" antihistamine Allegra. Six months later the FDA pulled Seldane off the market. Now it was up to Hoescht to "market Allegra . . . aggressively" as the *New York Times* reported, and reclaim its lost market share.[60]

But how to do it? Hoescht attempted to advertise Allegra on television, but to sidestep FDA requirements the company's Allegra ads never mentioned what the drug was for. The commercials featured a woman inexplicably windsurfing across a field of wheat, as the *Washington Post* reported. The ads were a disaster, mystifying consumers and providing ample fodder for late-night comedy shows.[61]

Then, in 1997, eight months after pulling Seldane, the FDA announced that TV drug ads would no longer have to portray the bad along with the good about new drugs. Instead, television ads could simply mention the very worst side effects, dispensing with the others by suggesting that consumers consult a Web site or call a 1-800 number to find out more. By allowing drugmakers to highlight the benefits of new drugs while sidelining drawbacks, the new rules would allow even marginally useful drugs, when promoted vigorously, to flourish.

"This is very good timing," enthused a Hoescht spokesperson.[62] Fall ragweed season was approaching. Now the company could run a proper ad campaign, reaching television's mass audiences with their message that Allegra was a better allergy drug than Claritin, better too than the cheap, over-the-counter remedies that many were opting for.

In 1997, Hoescht spent over $50 million advertising Allegra directly to consumers. It was money well spent; Allegra sales promptly doubled. Schering-Plough responded with over $74 million in consumer advertising for Claritin.[63] As the televised war between the antihistamines raged, Americans flocked to their doctors clamoring for Claritin and Allegra scrips. In the first eight months of 1998, "patient visits to doctors increased 2 percent, [but] visits for allergies rose five times as fast," the *New York Times* reported.[64] By 1999, drugmakers were spending more on hyping prescription antihistamines to consumers than any other class of drugs.[65]

And yet, a 2002 study that compared Zyrtec, Claritin, Allegra, and other nonsedating antihistamines found no differences in their efficacy. "When choosing a drug . . . for treatment of allergic rhinitis," the authors concluded, "the preference of the patients might be the one most important factor, because all the new histamine H_1-antagonists appear to be comparable in their efficacy."[66]

According to drug industry spokespeople and the FDA, the new "direct-to-consumer" advertising craze helped patients get the drugs they needed. "You need to be told by someone that those products are out there or you'll never know," FDA medical director Robert Temple said to the *Washington Post* in 1997.[67] As for health care providers, the new obsession for prescription allergy meds was hard to fathom. "Except for antibiotics," commented Mark DiGiorgio, a disgusted HMO executive, "we are spending more money on runny noses than anything else."[68]

The FDA's relaxation of drug advertising rules did much more than relieve Hoescht's business troubles. In the past, in order to build a market for a new prescription drug, the medical community would first have to be convinced of the necessity of the treatment. The doc-as-gatekeeper served as a skeptical check on drug companies that might try to sell a risky or useless drug. Now drug companies could reach consumers directly with their exhortations to get checked for dangerous new conditions and ask their doctors for brand-name drugs—and not just for medical problems, either, but for social problems, even for cosmetic ones. Soon scores of consumers whom most physicians would deem healthy were exposing themselves to the risks of pharmaceutical products, further diminishing the risk-benefit ratio of new drugs.

One such product is Viagra, launched by Pfizer in 1998. Pfizer was about to abandon sildenafil, a failed angina drug, when they picked up on its effect on men's erections. The company soon ran trials among men who had been impotent for five years or more. The drug appeared to overcome impotence in 70 to 80 percent of test subjects.[69] According to the NIH-funded Massachusetts Male Aging Study, started in 1987, over half of the thousands of forty-to-seventy-year-old men it surveyed had endured an episode or two of failed erections over the previous six months, but only about 10 percent suffered complete erectile dysfunction. Most of these cases were among men who had other health problems—they were older, tended to smoke, were overweight, and had high blood pressure.[70] Many such men could be expected to be taking medications such as nitrates and beta-blockers, prescribed to millions for angina and high blood pressure; for them, sildenafil could be downright dangerous. Quitting smoking, changing medication regimens, counseling, exercise, and weight loss, moreover, could safely relieve many of the less severe problems.[71]

And yet it was true, as Pfizer's marketing director put it, that "most men who are 45 or 47 don't have the same erections they had when they were 18."[72] These men, with a little help from Pfizer, could be convinced they had a treatable disease. In a prominent television ad campaign featuring no less respectable a personage than former senator Bob Dole, Pfizer announced that "erectile dysfunction (ED)," an obscure medical term dusted off to serve as a more palatable euphemism for impotence, was a serious medical condition that afflicted no fewer than thirty million American men.[73] It was, as one executive explained, "brilliant branding." "And it's not just about branding the drug; it's branding the condition and, by inference, a branding of the patient. . . . We're creating patient populations just as we're creating medicines, to make sure that products become blockbusters."[74] The vast majority of ED's supposed thirty million sufferers—about 80 percent—suffered only mild to moderate dysfunction, some as little as one episode of erection loss over the previous six months.[75]

Pfizer defended what critics would later call disease mongering by saying that they were raising awareness about a shameful disease. Many men "really do want to go to their doctors but can't imagine bringing it up," Pfizer's marketing director for Viagra, Janice Lipsky, said to the *New York Times* in 2004.[76] And yet, there was little evidence of any reluctance to seek out Viagra prescriptions. In Britain, for example, diagnoses of erectile dysfunction doubled.[77] By 1999, five million men had been prescribed Viagra, bringing in $1 billion in sales for Pfizer.[78] Treatment rates for erectile dysfunction soared above other conditions. In heart disease, by way of contrast, only one-third of patients who could benefit from aspirin are prescribed it by their physicians.[79]

The drug was obviously being used by people who had no impairment whatsoever. As *Playboy*'s Hugh Hefner put it, "It's more than an impotence drug: It's a recreational drug. It eliminates the boundaries between expectation and reality."[80] Almost immediately upon its launch, Viagra pills were making the rounds among thrill seekers at dance clubs and sex parties.[81] Nervous men used the drug for "date protection," feminist sex expert Leonore Tiefer scoffed. In Taiwan, a campaigning politician distributed the drug for free. In France, restaurants served "beef piccata in Viagra sauce."[82] If any needy men had somehow escaped a Viagra prescription, Wrigley planned to deliver the drug in an even more appealing form: Viagra-imbued chewing gum.[83]

The FDA logged over one hundred deaths linked to Viagra within the eight months following the drug's appearance on the market, suggesting that the drug may have been implicated in between two thousand and ten thousand deaths. (Between 1 percent and 5 percent of adverse effects of drugs are estimated to be reported to the FDA.) "My husband was 65 with several medical problems and taking several other drugs, but he got the same dose as an 18-year-old," complained the widow of one Viagra casualty.[84]

Regardless, like Prozac and Mevacor before it, Viagra paved the way for a $23 billion "life-enhancing" drug market—drugs designed not to heal the sick but rather to make the well feel better.[85] Prozac had established a $12 billion market for antidepressants. Mevacor founded a $10 billion market for cholesterol-lowering drugs, a market that grew by over 33 percent every year between 1987 and 1992.[86]

Rival companies predictably jockeyed to muscle into the new markets. But rather than improve upon the trailblazing blockbuster (or trying to improve upon it, failing, and marching forward anyway), many simply resorted to selling copycats. Between 1998 and 2002 "me-too" drugs—those deemed by regulators to offer no advantage over already available drugs—accounted for three-quarters of the new drugs approved by the FDA.[87]

Not only would the task of developing, testing, and reviewing the copycat drugs further burden already strained health care and regulatory systems, they would intensify the onslaught of drug marketing to dizzying heights. By 1998, drug companies were spending between two and three times more on marketing and administration than they did on research,[88] forking over no less than $1.3 billion on advertising directly to consumers.[89] The intense marketing says something about the drugs, former *New England Journal of Medicine* editor Marcia Angell says. "Truly good drugs don't have to be promoted very much. . . . Wouldn't the world beat a path to the door of a company that produced, say, a cure for cancer?" Me-too drugs, on the other hand, "require relentless flogging, because companies need to persuade doctors and the public that there is some reason to prescribe one instead of another."[90]

Rather than improving upon Mevacor, for example, drug companies launched a plethora of copycat statins. Four years after launching Mevacor, Merck introduced its cousin, simvastatin (Zocor). That same year Bristol-Myers Squibb released its pravastatin (Pravachol). Pfizer soon offered atorvastatin (Lipitor), followed by Bayer's cerivastatin (Baycol) and AstraZeneca's rosuvastatin (Crestor).[91]

The abundance of statins stood in direct contrast to their slender benefits, especially for the millions of Americans who weren't at especially high risk for heart disease. According to one analysis, more than four hundred people with mild cholesterol would need to be treated with statin drugs in order to prevent a single coronary heart disease event,[92] a success rate that pales in comparison to improved diet and exercise regimes. After all, half of all heart attacks occur in people who have normal cholesterol levels.[93]

Statin makers were forced to exaggerate, with all the problematic public health effects that would follow: "You may think you're healthy," Pfizer ads warned, over tragic scenes of middle-aged men dramatically collapsing midmeal, "but too much cholesterol in your blood can cause a heart attack."[94] With all the competition in the already crowded field AstraZeneca lavished a $1 billion advertising budget on Crestor.[95]

One way drug companies could distinguish their otherwise indistinguishable me-too drugs was by tinkering with the dose. At lower doses the prescription antihistamines effected more marketable claims—they were less sedating, albeit also, it seemed, less effective. In fact, in the RCTs of Claritin submitted for FDA approval, the drug appeared only marginally better than nothing at all: in one trial Claritin affected a 46 percent improvement compared to 35 percent on placebo. According to an allergist on the FDA advisory committee that considered the drug, at the dose that Schering wanted to sell it, Claritin "is not very different than placebo clinically." A larger dose might be more effective but would make patients drowsy, undermining the one marketing claim that set the drug apart from its much cheaper over-the-counter alternatives. Schering wasn't interested.[96] In statin drugs higher doses led to better marketing claims. At higher doses statins could reduce cholesterol levels more rapidly and severely, allowing drugmakers to claim their statins were "more effective" and "easier to prescribe" than alternative statins. The trouble, critics complained, was that the higher and one-size-fits-all doses added diminishingly little more effectiveness while significantly increasing the risk of adverse events, such as rhabdomyolysis (the potentially fatal break-down of muscle fibers).[97] All of the statin drugs cause rhabdomyolysis to some degree, a factoid that generally emerged after the drugs hit pharmacy shelves. The problem was so bad with Bayer's statin Baycol—based on the number of deaths reported, it appears that over six hundred people may have been killed by the drug[98]—that it was withdrawn after a few years on the market. The latest competitor, AstraZeneca's Crestor (launched in 2004), is being sold at an even higher dose than the other statins, and triggered cases of rhabdomyolysis even before the FDA approved it.[99]

While consumers replaced doctors as the originating sources for new drug prescriptions, physicians' ability to judge new drugs independently weakened. The pressure on doctors to liberally dole out prescriptions for the new blockbuster drugs is intense. Drug company dollars have penetrated nearly every corner of medicine, from medical school to hospital corridors and continuing medical education courses, where they bombard physicians with positive information about new drugs, free samples, and luxurious perks for the biggest prescribers.

Exposés of doctors accepting elaborate resort vacations and free concert tickets from drug companies grab headlines, but the more run-of-the-mill drug marketing, in which boosterism masquerades as research and education, typically goes unreported. For example, nine out of ten physicians rely on the *Physicians' Desk Reference* for information about which drugs to prescribe.[100] The *PDR*, delivered free of charge to all practicing physicians in the country and updated annually, presents itself as a useful, unbiased reference book. In fact, the *PDR* is funded by drug companies, and the book itself is simply an alphabetical compendium of drug companies' product labels.[101] If research not funded by the industry reveals that a drug is ineffective, dangerous, or redundant, doctors who rely on the *PDR* would never know it, as such information is excluded from the *PDR* (unless the FDA orders a label change). Nor are independent drug reference books able to compete against the *PDR*. The well-regarded *AMA Drug Evaluations*, for example, sputtered along on less than twenty thousand copies worth of sales every year before admitting defeat and ceasing publication in 1996.[102]

In many states medical boards themselves encourage doctors to participate in drug company–sponsored seminars and workshops. Thirty-four states require that doctors participate in continuing medical education (CME) programs every year in order to maintain their licenses to practice. More than half of the cost of these programs are now paid by drug companies. Their intent is not to teach doctors about the pros and cons of new drug therapies, or to advocate nondrug solutions to medical problems. They are instead openly regarded as marketing opportunities. "Medical education is a powerful tool that can deliver your message," one CME company announced to drug companies.[103] Industry-sponsored CME programs work, too: one study, comparing outcomes among heart attack patients in states with CME requirements and those without found little difference between the two—save for the fact that patients in CME states were "significantly more likely to receive brands of thrombolytic . . . drugs manufactured by drug companies that often sponsor CME events," as *Heart Disease Weekly* reported in 2004.[104]

If all that wasn't sufficient, drug companies often resort to simply paying doctors to prescribe their drugs. Thousands of practicing physicians are enticed into switching their patients to new drugs through industry-sponsored postmarketing "trials." For these putative trials companies find physicians who are most likely to prescribe their new drug, and pay them hundreds or even thousands of dollars for "enrolling" patients in the "study" of the new drug. The idea is to entice doctors and patients into trying a new drug in the hope that they'll continue the prescription after the trial ends, this time at top dollar. "Make no mistake about it," announced one industry marketing memo. "The . . . study is the single most important sales initiative. . . . [I]f at least

20,000 of the 25,000 patients involved in the study remain on [the drug], it could mean up to a $10,000,000 boost in sales."[105]

As doctors' prestige and salaries nosedive under managed care, drug companies lavish them with free vacations, dinners, reference books, and drug samples. The billions spent on direct-to-consumer marketing had patients asking for drugs by name. Was it really surprising then, that when Americans visited their doctors, two out or three times they'd come home with a new prescription or a free drug sample?[106]

As each check and balance on the drug industry—rigorous regulation, fairly informed consumers, skeptical physicians—fell by the wayside, so too did the independence of academic medical researchers, who could easily destroy the marketing goliath that the blockbuster drug industry has become. Just as a *60 Minutes* exposé or a scathing *Consumer Reports* review could destroy the sales of other dubious products, a single study exposing the overblown claims of drug marketers, published in a prestigious medical journal like the *New England Journal of Medicine* or *JAMA*, could devastate a new drug.

Fortunately for the industry, though, by the mid-1990s the handful of independent medical researchers who investigated the veracity of drug industry marketing claims were "an endangered species facing extinction," according to the NIH. Enchanted by the dazzling promise of the new genetics revolution—so-called basic research based in laboratories—NIH funding for the messy work of experimenting on humans had dried up, dropping to just one-tenth of the NIH's extramural budget.[107]

It was either take drug company money or perish, many academic researchers felt. The drug industry, by 1995, was spending nearly 40 percent more than the government did on medical research.[108] "For academic medicine not to avail itself of the resources of the pharmaceutical industry and private sector would be foolish," said University of North Carolina psychiatry professor Jeffrey

Lieberman to the *Wall Street Journal*. "It would be like major sports saying they won't take advertising from Nike."[109]

And so, academic medical researchers under industry contracts cranked out a steady stream of positive research detailing minor differences between nearly identical drugs. According to one analysis, 95 percent of industry-sponsored studies of cancer drugs rendered favorable results as opposed to just 62 percent of those funded by nonprofits. "Is academic medicine for sale?" wondered the *New England Journal of Medicine*'s then editor Marcia Angell in a May 2000 editorial.[110] "No," came the response from one cynic. "The current owner is very happy with it."[111]

Drug companies retorted that they conducted the exacting randomized controlled trials that the FDA's regulations required. The model's integrity is unassailable, no matter who implements it, they argued. Experts in the field, by and large, agreed.[112] And yet, there is wiggle room in RCTs. They are ill equipped to find answers to questions they don't ask. What's more, they can be subtly manipulated to make new drugs look better than they are. A new drug might be pitted against a lower dose of its competitor drug, or against an inferior form of it. The majority of trials comparing Pfizer's fluconazole to amphotericin B, for example, administered the amphotericin orally, even though that drug works better intravenously. Or new drugs might be tested in subjects much heartier than those who would end up swallowing the meds later on, lessening side effects. For example, arthritis-drug makers fill over 97 percent of the spots in their trials with subjects under sixty-five years of age, despite the fact that most of the patients who will be prescribed the drugs are elderly.[113]

Despite such hijinks, occasionally industry-sponsored academics come up with results that don't jibe with a company's marketing message. By and large such studies are squelched and the academics sacked. A few months of data might be dropped, for example, or a study might be redesigned to render a more pleasing result. Academics who don't go along with the game risk being slapped with lawsuits. "Companies can play hardball," complained Wake Forest University public health professor Curt Furberg, MD. "Many investigators can't play hardball back."[114]

Bruce Psaty, one the nation's leading cardiovascular researchers, saw firsthand just how.[115] During the 1990s Psaty undertook a study funded by the National Heart, Blood, and Lung Institute, looking into the differences between patients who took various popular calcium channel blocker drugs for their high blood pressure and those who didn't. At the time around six million Americans were prescribed calcium channel blockers, but few long-term studies had been conducted on their safety.[116]

This was precisely the kind of research that the drug industry would be loath to take on: a study that pitted rival drugs in a head-to-head comparison. And Psaty's findings were exactly the kind of results that drug companies would be loath to hear. According to his study, contrary to drugmakers' marketing messages, the most popular drugs increased the risk of a heart attack by about 60 percent (from 10 in 1,000 to 16 in 1,000).[117] With millions of people taking the heavily marketed drugs, the increased risk was a significant public health concern.

The results were quickly picked up by the Associated Press and other media outlets. Panic ensued. Hundreds of calls from distraught patients, doctors, and drug companies poured in to Psaty's office, forcing him to hire extra help. Doctors and industry execs were irate, calling Psaty's report alarmist. "This is a great example of news that's not ready for prime time," seethed the American Heart Association's Rodman Starke.[118]

While *Pharmaceutical Executive* magazine pooh-poohed Psaty's findings—"many people who die are taking some drugs," the magazine noted breezily[119]—Pfizer demanded that Psaty's university submit mountains of notes, meeting minutes, and records for their review. Drug maufacturers criticized Psaty's study and, he says, publicly questioned his integrity. The embattled Psaty and other similarly harassed researchers aired their sad story in a

1997 *New England Journal of Medicine* paper, under the headline "The messenger under attack."[120]

By 2000, the proportion of the nation's health care budget devoted to drugs was growing by 15 percent every year—almost twice the rate of growth in spending for hospitals and doctors—and was expected to continue to rise over the coming decade.[121] While the industry takes pains to point out how this outlay of cash actually saves society money, by preventing costly hospitalizations, in fact most of the increased spending on drugs centered around just a handful of heavily marketed, brand-name drugs—not much more than two dozen of the over nine thousand drugs on the market. The bestsellers included such nakedly commercial hits as Astra-Zeneca's acid-reflux drug Nexium, which contains the same active molecule as the off-patent drug that preceded it, Prilosec, and allergy drug Clarinex, the metabolite of its off-patent parent drug Claritin.[122]

Clearly, the relentless growth of the drug industry—and the concomitant expansion of its clinical research activities—are not inevitable results of the American quest for good health. According to the World Health Organization, of the thousands of drugs available in the United States, just over three hundred are essential for public health. That's not to say that such new drugs aren't useful to some subset of patients, as FDA officials and industry execs often point out. "The availability of me-too drugs can reduce health care costs," says former FDA commissioner Mark McClellan. "If there is just one cholesterol medication available, the price may be very high; if there are three or four or five, the price can come down a lot."[123] Plus, each patient's unique physiology responds differently to subtly different drugs—when one statin doesn't work, perhaps another will. And even hyped lifestyle drugs like Viagra have important medical uses, not just by treating those who genuinely suffer from erectile dysfunction, but by counteracting sexual side effects brought on by the treatment of more serious diseases. Drugs that come in tasty syrups, convenient pills, and handy nasal sprays help more people take the medicines they need.

But the number of people helped—and the margin by which they are healed—is certainly narrow, and the flip side of the mass marketing of blockbuster drugs is a heavy toll in adverse effects that would otherwise remain sporadic. Today, when elderly patients are rushed to the emergency room, it is 50 percent more likely that their problem stems from taking too many drugs, rather than from not taking enough.[124] Approved drugs kill over one hundred thousand Americans every year,[125] not counting the scores whose bad reactions are unreported or wrongly attributed to the disease the drug is meant to treat,[126] making adverse reactions to pill popping the fifth leading cause of death in the United States.[127]

Each new drug must be tested on scores of warm bodies, a "conditional privilege" that society grants to investigators because it values medical innovation and beneficial new drugs, as the NIH notes in its 2004 *Guidelines for the Conduct of Research Involving Human Subjects*.[128]

And yet, what the recent history of our drug development and marketing system shows is that there is no easy equation between new drugs and health benefits, not even in the United States, where people consume more new drugs than anywhere else in the world. This is as true for me-too ED drugs that lead drug company sales as the masses of drugs aimed at more serious illnesses that comprise the majority of industry portfolios. For, although the risks to experimental subjects in a trial for me-too lifestyle drugs aren't insignificant, they are generally short-term trials involving subjects who are not seriously ill. In drugs aimed at more dangerous conditions, the contrast between the risk-shouldering subjects and the distant beneficiaries can be stark indeed.

4

Uncaging the Guinea Pig

Long before the drug industry embarked on its global hunt for bodies in the poor reaches of the world, Western medical researchers relied on the bodies of their own vulnerable populations to satisfy their scientific curiosity.

The notion of manipulating human bodies to answer scientific questions arose, in part, in recognition of the fact that even the most elaborate pharmacopoeias did little to muffle the death toll from disease and infection. For countless bloody centuries nobody really knew how the body functioned or why it became diseased. The circulating blood, the pumping heart, the pulsating nerves and organs: none of these hidden mechanisms had revealed themselves, and the body remained as mysterious as the strange factors that suddenly appeared to sicken it.[1]

But by dissecting bodies and looking inside them, Western physicians began to figure out how they functioned and what went wrong when they became infirm. Over a thousand years human dissections and vivisections—the mutilation of live human beings—slowly revealed the body's mechanisms. Most of the cutting took place on the bodies of the poor and imprisoned, doubling as public spectacle and social opprobrium.[2]

The travails of those who ended up as "clinical material" rarely surfaced in polite company. Poor and colored people were generally considered less sensitive to pain anyway. As the prominent French physiologist and avid dissector Claude Bernard wrote in his 1865 *Introduction to the Study of Experimental Medicine*, scientists considered themselves immune to the "cries of people of fashion" along with those of the dissected themselves.[3] Medical science was above the fray, he insisted, and could only be judged by its own practitioners. As for the human subjects involved, if society didn't respect their rights, why should scientists?

Such attitudes persisted uncontested for nearly a century. It was a government-sponsored inquiry into the course of syphilis that would finally expose them to a shocked public.

Syphilis is an old American disease, brought back to Europe by Columbus's returning sailors. In some people, the corkscrew-shaped *Treponema* bacteria causes no symptoms for years; some even naturally rid their body of it without ever knowing they've had it, inadvertently passing it on to others through sexual contact. For an unlucky minority the bacterium causes serious disease. It begins with genital sores, then a general rash and ulceration, and finally "revolting abscesses eating into bones and destroying the nose, lips, and genitals," as medical historian Roy Porter described it. Untreated, it often proves fatal. (To repair the damage to syphilitics' noses, sixteenth-century surgeons sewed flaps of skin from the upper arm onto their faces, leaving them to recover, arm attached to nose, for weeks at a time.) Medicine had little to offer. Until the synthesis of arsenic-based drugs in 1908, physicians prescribed the application of mercury ointments, a useless therapy that nevertheless caused teeth to fall out, ulcers to form on the gums, and bones to crumble.[4]

The economic burden of the disease weighed heavily in the U.S. South of the 1920s. The contagion ran rampant among the impoverished black laborers that many industries relied upon. If those sick with syphilis could be somehow treated, "the results would more than pay for the cost in better labor efficiency," as one doctor from the U.S. Public Health Service (PHS) pointed out. Medical research into the field was urgent.[5]

With its potent whiff of sex, disfigurement, and death trailing behind, syphilis was considered an illicit, dirty disease. Syphilitics were so despised that during the 1930s U.S. hospitals refused to treat them. In 1934 a U.S. government health commissioner was kicked off the radio for simply uttering the word "syphilis" on the air. Sufferers of venereal diseases were relegated to special clinics, where their immoral ways couldn't contaminate the upstanding sick in nearby hospitals. Their fates in the clinics couldn't have been heartening. By then, standard treatment—over a year of painful weekly injections of arsenic—was expensive, time consuming, and only partially effective.[6]

Public disgust for syphilitics made experimentation easier in many ways. In 1931, Rockefeller-funded malaria researcher Mark Boyd injected the *Plasmodium falciparum* malarial parasite into black patients demented with syphilis at a Florida hospital. True, the idea of killing the syphilis bacterium by inducing high malarial fevers was a therapeutic craze at the time. But while white patients were generally administered the mild *Plasmodium vivax* malarial parasite, Boyd infected his black subjects with the parasite's deadly cousin *falciparum*. No law or social mores required that he ask for the patients' or their families' consent, although he did do so for the eventual autopsies of the patients' bodies.[7]

In 1929, a Public Health Service feasibility study determined that a mass treatment program for rural black workers suffering from syphilis was possible. But by 1932, funding for such elaborate endeavors had dried up, and the government doctors' attention turned from providing care to scientific research. What if they enrolled syphilis-infected patients into a study, provided no treatment at all, and just watched what happened? Several interesting questions might be answered, maintained the PHS's Dr. Taliaferro Clark, who conceived of the study. Perhaps the course of the disease was different in blacks than in whites, for instance, or perhaps no treatment was better than treatment. Whatever the case, autopsies of subjects who succumbed to the disease while under the researchers' watch could help shed light on these pressing questions.[8]

Even back then such a "natural history" study would likely have been impossible to conduct on white, literate, or middle-class patients. But the subjects for this study would be impoverished, mostly illiterate black male sharecroppers in Macon County, Alabama, around the town of Tuskegee, where syphilis rates were soaring.

American science already relied on blacks as a source of clinical material, just as American plantations relied on them for their back-breaking labors in the field. The black janitors and technicians who cleaned up after American scientists were often called upon to supply animal and human bodies to experiment on. Young black boys could be enticed into capturing and etherizing dogs for experiments, and black men to tend experimental animals in the dark corridors of research hospitals; either could be approached to offer their bodies for ghastly experiments, such as one in which subjects had to swallow a twelve-foot-long tube that would be inflated later while lodged deep in the body.[9]

Still, the government doctors found recruitment for their no-treatment syphilis study difficult, even among the black workers they derided as ignorant and lazy in private correspondence later collected by Wellesley medical historian Susan Reverby. Finally, they resorted to deception, offering what they called "free treatment." Nearly four hundred black male sharecroppers who considered themselves ill with "bad blood," but who in fact were suffering from late-stage syphilis, along with 201 healthy black men who would serve as controls, enrolled in the study. As the subjects were unaware that they suffered from syphilis, the government doctors were under no pressure to offer the standard syphilis treatments of the time. They gave, instead, the long-dismissed mercury ointments, along with aspirin, tonics, free lunches, and burial insurance, watching and taking notes as the condition of the syphilitic men worsened. As it was imperative that the patients in the study not be treated with any medicines, which would contaminate the resulting syphilitic corpse, the government doctors met with local clinicians "to ask their cooperation in not treating the men," according to a researcher involved in the study.[10]

Deceived and untreated, the sick men considered themselves lucky to be involved in the study. "The ride to and from the hospital in this vehicle with the Government emblem on the front door, chauffeured by a nurse, was a mark of distinction for many of the men who enjoyed waving to their neighbors as they drove by," the nurse recruited to entice the men into the study recalled. Believing themselves graced with free medical care from government doctors, they started families, unknowingly spreading the infection to their partners and children.[11]

The government doctors felt under no obligation to conceal the deception at the heart of their research from their colleagues. After all, in the mid-1930s, medical research was the stuff of heroic drama. A polio victim, Franklin Delano Roosevelt, sat in the White House, urging Americans to send in their spare change to support medical research into polio. In 1936, a blockbuster film, *The Story of Louis Pasteur*, extolled the field's forefather. No notion that research subjects might require protections from the ministrations of their doctor scientists, or that black people might be entitled to the same rights and freedoms as whites, existed to counterbalance the prerogative of researchers to do what they may. When the doctors busy at Tuskegee presented their preliminary findings at the annual meeting of the American Medical Association (AMA) that year, noting that the patients from whom they purposely withheld treatment were getting sicker much faster than their controls, nobody batted an eye. Papers about the study appeared in the medical literature at about five-year intervals from then on.[12]

With the arrival of penicillin in the 1940s, and its remarkable efficiency in treating syphilis, the nontreatment study in Tuskegee lost its primary reason for being. What was the point in seeing how the disease progressed without treatment, when treatment was now so simple and effective? Yet the Public Health Service clung to its original plan. They did not offer penicillin to the hundreds of black men under their care suffering from syphilis. On the contrary, in order to protect the integrity of their data, they conspired with local draft boards to withhold the army's standard syphilis treatment from any Tuskegee subjects drafted into service.[13]

After all, medical progress required risk-taking, and sometimes researchers had to employ trickery or exploit their authority over vulnerable subjects in order to get the job done. In 1943, as the country headed to war, the U.S. Public Health Service paid two hundred prisoners one hundred dollars each to be infected with gonorrhea as government doctors watched, hoping to learn about its transmission. In another study government scientists infected eight hundred prisoners and hospital patients with malaria to study the efficacy of new antimalarial drugs. In that study the docs placed malaria-infected mosquitoes on prisoners' warm stomachs as a *Life* magazine photographer hovered nearby.[14]

As documented by University of Virginia bioethicist Jonathan D. Moreno in his 2000 book on secret state experiments, *Undue Risk*, thousands of American soldiers were used in experiments designed to determine the fatal dose of poison gas, which had felled scores in World War I. In one test, termed a trial of "summer clothing," soldiers were locked into gas chambers full of mustard gas in exchange for a three-day pass. Wearing only street clothes and a gas mask, some pleaded with their captors to be released but were denied until falling unconscious.[15]

Starting in 1946, scientists working with the Atomic Energy Commission (later renamed the Nuclear Regulatory Commission) launched a series of studies involving human consumption of radioactive materials at two schools for troubled children in Massachusetts, Fernald and Wrentham. The child inmates at these brutal institutions were heavily tranquilized, and were consigned half naked to bare, cement-floored rooms outfitted with grates into which their urine and feces could be hosed. Scientists fed the children meals contaminated with radioactive material, drawing their blood afterward to study how their bodies fared.

The children were so neglected, as one resident subject remembered years later, that they "would do practically anything for attention." Even so, their parents had to be actively misled in order for the experiments to proceed. In letters to the parents the studies were presented as "examinations" on nutrition, aimed at "brighter children" who would receive "special diets" as part of their membership in a special "Science Club." The Fernald and Wrentham studies continued until 1973, with periodic reports appearing in medical journals.[16]

While the government pursued these inquiries in order to further their political and military goals, university scientists signed on for a chance to enter the exciting new field of radiation experimentation. As one prominent scientist remembered, "This was something like bacteriology . . . this was going to be a terrific field."[17] In a 1945 study eighteen hospitalized patients under the care of physicians from the University of Rochester, the University of Chicago, and the University of California were secretly injected with plutonium. The purpose was to discern how the body processed the metal, and researchers pored over their plutonium-injected patients' urine and stools and sampled their extracted teeth to find out. Patients were told that the doctors' pointed and ongoing interest in them had nothing to do with experimentation but was part and parcel of their "long-term care," as Moreno writes. Some were even dug up from their graves to see how much plutonium remained in their bones; their families were told this was in order to discern the effects of "past medical treatment."[18]

Similar state experimentation proceeded in other Western countries. In Australia, over eight hundred Jewish refugees and injured soldiers were purposely infected with malaria, sometimes at doses equal to the bites of thirteen thousand infected mosquitoes. The government scientists withheld antimalarial treatment from their shivering charges while they removed up to two pints of blood and injected them with insulin and adrenalin in order to simulate blood loss, starvation, and anxiety. "They never told us anything," recalls one subject who survived the trial. "At first

I didn't realize it was dangerous. . . . I thought it would be an adventure and that is why I went," recalled another.[19]

Physicians in Fascist Germany and imperial Japan likewise performed nontherapeutic experiments, but in their cases, subjects were condemned to death regardless of the results. Japanese scientists injected their Chinese prisoners with plague, cholera, and other pathogens, slaughtering them when they finally became too weak to provide any interesting data. They also conducted "field tests" on unsuspecting Chinese villages, poisoning more than one thousand wells with typhoid bacilli, releasing plague-infested rats and spraying typhus and cholera on wheat fields.[20]

During World War II Nazi scientists conducted a range of grisly experiments on concentration camp inmates. Eager to understand how the human body functioned at high altitudes, they encased subjects in decompression chambers, pumped all the air out, and then dissected the subjects while still alive to study their lungs. To see firsthand the effects of dehydration they starved subjects and forced them to drink only saltwater. They injected children with gasoline. They removed their subjects' bones and limbs, many dying from infections after their useless surgeries, others simply being shot. Inmates were injected with phenol to see how long it would take them to die.[21]

Prisoners were used, a Nazi officer later explained, because "volunteers could not very well be expected, as the experiments could be fatal."[22]

The Nazi regime's medical research program fell under scrutiny soon after the war ended. Some twenty Nazi doctors of the hundreds or more who may have been involved in Germany's wartime experimentation were selected to stand trial before the International Military Tribunal, set up in Nuremberg by the United States and the rest of the victorious allies.[23]

Though the U.S. government's own deceptive and exploitative wartime experiments would not see the light of day for nearly fifty years,[24] it still wasn't easy for the Americans to prove that their medical research was substantively different from that of the

Nazis. Each submerged the interests of human subjects in order to procure scientific data.

The defendants argued that their wartime experiments were essentially run-of-the-mill medical research, "the logical expression of the values of German medical science," as University of California historian Anita Guerrini notes in her 2003 book, *Experimenting with Humans and Animals*. The subjects were volunteers, they said, who were scheduled to be killed anyway. And their suffering had to be balanced against the benefits the research would bestow upon others. That is, "it was legitimate that a few should have been made to suffer for the good of the many," Guerrini wrote.[25] Wasn't this the guiding philosophy of all Western medical research? Hadn't American doctors purposely given prisoners a fatal disease in their own experiments? the Nazis' defense lawyers asked the court, reciting from the 1945 *Life* magazine article on the government's prisoner-malaria experiments.[26]

To uphold the reputation of American medical research, the prosecution called upon its star medical ethics expert, the University of Illinois's Andrew Ivy, MD. The fact was, though, that nobody in the American medical research establishment had questioned the ethics of the prisoner-malaria experiments when the *Life* spread appeared in 1945. Nobody had said anything in 1946, when PHS doctors had reported that their untreated patients at Tuskegee were dying at nearly twice the rate as their healthy controls. The truth was, while the Hippocratic oath guided medical practice no American medical researcher was bound by any written ethical principles.[27]

Nazi medical experimentation may have fallen into a lower category of depravity than what was happening in the United States, conducted as it was in the context of wholesale butchery, but the fact was that little could be called upon to prove this was so, at least not without knocking the medical research establishment off its pedestal. Ivy was forced to act quickly. As the trial progressed he convened a panel to investigate the prisoner-malaria experiments and wrote up some ethical principles to govern human experimentation, presenting his draft to the American Medical Association. Ivy represented his hastily improvised solutions, yet to be considered by the AMA, as "the basic principles approved by the American Medical Association for the use of human beings as subjects in medical experiments." He also presented his newly formed panel on the prisoner-malaria experiments as an ongoing one, though it had yet to meet even once. If the public's high regard for medical research were any guide, it should have been easy to prove Nazi medical research worse than America's, but the country's leading medical ethics expert had to perjure himself in order to do it.[28]

In the end, four Nazi doctors were hanged after their trial at Nuremberg and eight were sentenced to prison. The rest, along with others who were not tried, returned home to their university jobs and medical practices.[29]

The judges, in their decision, issued a new set of ethical guidelines to govern medical experiments. These would become known weightily as the Nuremberg Code, but in fact were mostly lifted directly from the few principles jotted down by Andrew Ivy.[30] The most pertinent of the ten principles was the first one: that human subjects in experiments should understand what they are getting into and agree to participate. Experimental subjects should not be powerless prisoners of war and the like either, but "so situated as to be able to exercise free power of choice." Experiments should only be conducted when absolutely necessary "so as to yield fruitful results for the good of society," and risks to subjects should be minimized by all means possible. Any dangers to the subjects must be outweighed by the "humanitarian importance of the problem to be solved by the experiment," and certainly should include none that researchers knew in advance might result in death or disability.[31]

The medical profession lauded the code publicly, but privately tended to dismiss it. Yale psychiatrist Jay Katz remembered his professors' reactions to the Nuremberg Code: "It was a good code for barbarians but an unnecessary code for ordinary physicians."[32]

And in any case, the new code was voluntary and vague. When the medical establishment used the code to consider whether a given experiment's potential social benefits outweighed definite risks to subjects living today, they were usually able to err on the side of the former. For example, in most countries the Nuremberg Code was interpreted to exclude prisoners from any kind of medical research. In the United States Ivy's committee found the government's prisoner-malaria experiments ethically "ideal," a view it announced in the February 14, 1948, issue of *JAMA*.[33]

During the 1950s and 1960s medical researchers continued to conduct experiments on powerless subjects that fell well short of Nuremberg's ideal of minimal risk and informed and voluntary consent. For example, in 1952 Jonas Salk conducted early trials of his experimental polio vaccine on mentally retarded children at the Polk State School in Pennsylvania; in many cases, only the state officials who were the legal guardians of the children gave permission. Between 1957 and 1960 another polio researcher, the drug industry–sponsored Hilary Koprowski likewise tested his polio vaccine on retarded children in New York, as well as on 325,000 children in what was then called the Belgian Congo.[34]

In other cases informed consent was skipped over entirely, for the experiments themselves were secret. Between 1944 and 1960 government researchers secretly released radioactive material over mostly Native American and Latino communities in order to determine how the material dispersed and its effects on human health. Likewise, in a series of experiments conducted between 1953 and 1957 medical researchers at Massachusetts General Hospital exposed eleven unsuspecting patients to uranium, hoping to find out how the substance might affect inadvertently exposed government workers.[35]

The doctrine of minimizing risks to test subjects was fuzzy enough to allow investigators to openly infect otherwise healthy people in order to see what might happen. For example, in a series of medical experiments between 1963 and 1966 New York University pediatrician Saul Krugman injected healthy children with hepatitis virus, a liver-infecting pathogen spread through fecal matter. Working at Willowbrook State School, a state-run institution for mentally retarded and other disabled children, Krugman's team obtained hepatitis-laden feces, centrifuged, heated, and treated it with antibiotics, and then mixed it with five parts of chocolate milk to one part of feces. They fed the contaminated concoction to uninfected children and tracked their deterioration. According to Krugman, purposely infecting the children didn't subject them to any great risk, because Willowbrook was rife with infectious diseases anyway.[36] This was a facility, after all, where inmates sometimes smeared the walls with feces.[37]

Krugman's Willowbrook studies went on until the 1970s, resulting in breakthroughs in hepatitis research that made Krugman a medical hero. He was awarded some of the most prestigious prizes in medicine.[38]

These transgressions only started to leak into public notice in the mid-1960s. First, in 1966, a Harvard anesthesiology professor named Henry K. Beecher described dozens of studies that violated Nuremberg standards in a *New England Journal of Medicine* paper, including one in which subjects in a typhoid study had been denied effective medication, leading to twenty-three deaths, and another in which ill patients had been purposely injected with live cancer cells. The following year, across the Atlantic, British physician Maurice Pappworth released his book *Human Guinea Pigs: Experimentation on Man*, likening the research practices of Western scientists to those of the Nazi doctors.[39]

Revelations from Beecher and Pappworth proved insufficiently persuasive to many investigators, including those continuing their inquiries in Tuskegee. Outraged letters to the Public Health Service about the study started to trickle in,[40] but when the Centers for Disease Control (CDC) reviewed the study in the late 1960s (responsibility for the program had transferred to that agency in 1957[41]), they nevertheless decided that it should continue until the

study's "endpoints" were reached, that is, until all of the ill subjects died. By 1969, untreated syphilis had felled up to hundred of
the subjects of the study. "You will never have another study like
this; take advantage of it," a CDC reviewer suggested.[42]

But with the 1960s-era articulation of the rights of blacks,
women, the poor, and other oppressed people, the racist paternal-
ism of the Tuskegee study could not remain submerged much
longer. One staffer in the Public Health Service, Peter J. Buxton,
felt that "what was being done was very close to murder and was,
if you will, an institutionalized form of murder," and he brought
his concerns to his superiors. After they delivered "a rather stern
lecture" about the benefits of the study, as Buxton recalled, he
brought the information to a reporter friend. In 1972, Jean Heller
reported on the Tuskegee Study of Untreated Syphilis in the *New
York Times* and unleashed a storm of outrage.[43]

Aided in part by revelations about Tuskegee, by the early 1970s
unalloyed faith in medicine stalled. The heralded new drugs and
medical techniques of the postwar era had ended up costing more
and producing less by way of better health than most had antici-
pated. Between 1962 and 1972 Americans' health care bill had
tripled; the cost of prescription drugs had doubled.[44] And yet,
Americans suffered higher infant mortality rates and lower life
expectancies than most Europeans. In January 1970 *Fortune* magazine asserted that American medicine "is inferior in quality,
wastefully dispensed, and inequitably financed. . . . Whether
poor or not, Americans are badly served by the obsolete, over-
strained medical system that has grown up around them helter-
skelter." The situation was so bad that even the business press had
come to sound like rabble-rousing activists. "The time has come
for radical change," *Fortune* opined.[45]

The Tuskegee study quickly achieved notoriety as a prime example of racist medical arrogance. Prominent physicians took up
their pens to decry what they called a "crime against humanity"

of "awesome dimensions." Senate hearings and a $1.8 billion law-suit followed.[46] By the time the Tuskegee study was finally termi-nated on November 16, 1972, the untreated Tuskegee subjects had unwittingly infected twenty-two women, seventeen children, and two grandchildren. The U.S. government agreed to pay $37,500 to each syphilitic patient who was still alive and $15,000 to those who served as controls.[47]

The Tuskegee revelations proved to the public the folly of al-lowing the moral integrity of scientists to suffice as protection for experimental subjects. Government needed to regulate the med-ical research industry just as they regulated mines and factories.

The National Research Act was passed in 1974, and an entirely new actor barged into the test clinic: independent oversight com-mittees. Under the act the integrity of informed consent, the min-imization of risks, and the breadth of data supporting the goals of the research would be assessed not by investigators themselves, but by independent committees empowered to ban or alter trials that didn't pass muster. These ethics committees, called institu-tional review boards (IRB) in the United States, would be the final arbiters on the ethics of human experiments.

The 1974 national commission convened to elaborate on ethical principles guiding human experimentation in the United States went further. According to its Belmont Report, scientists had to practice "respect for persons," "beneficence," and something even more ambitious: justice. Experiments should not be conducted on the impoverished, incarcerated, and other vulnerable populations solely for the benefit of the rich and free, or to sate the curiosity of researchers.[48]

These ethical obligations echoed those articulated in another voluntary code then making the rounds. In 1975, the United States along with thirty-four other countries signed onto the "Declaration of Helsinki," a bold document crafted by the World Medical Asso-ciation, a group representing dozens of national physicians' organ-izations from around the globe. The declaration urged voluntary informed consent, the use of independent ethics committees, and that investigators prioritize their subjects' well-being above all other concerns, including "the interests of science and society." In the interests of justice, the declaration suggested, research subjects should be assured of access to the best health interventions identified in the study, and that their societies enjoy a "reasonable likelihood" of benefiting from the results of the experiment.[49]

Over the following years the new ethical principles developed in Belmont and Helsinki slowly trickled into the federal regulations governing clinical research in the United States. These regulations bound all research on American subjects and applied as well to any researchers accepting U.S. government funding no matter where they conducted their experiments.

Any drug company hankering for FDA approval to market new drugs would have to abide by the new regulations too—unless they conducted their trials outside the United States without alerting the FDA first. In that case, according to FDA rules, the Declaration of Helsinki (or local laws, whichever afforded more protection) would suffice.[50]

Between World War II and the mid-1970s regulators had arduously built a wall, brick by brick, to protect the human rights and dignity of human research subjects from the inquisitive investigators itching for access to them. The first major assault on these barriers came not long afterward. Propelled by the spread of HIV in the darkest days of the AIDS pandemic, the medical research establishment rushed the wall, and found it a challenging but not insurmountable hurdle.

5

HIV and the Second-rate Solution

From the Nazi camps to Tuskegee, when investigators needed their test subjects to suffer in order to acquire results, they often assumed the posture of the innocent bystander: in the concentration camps, inmates were going to be killed anyway; at Willowbrook, the children would have infected themselves with hepatitis if the scientists hadn't intervened; at Tuskegee, the sharecroppers wouldn't have been able to afford treatment, so what did it matter that investigators didn't provide any?

According to the new ethics regime established in the 1970s, such rationalizations would no longer be sufficient. According to Helsinki, "considerations related to the well-being of the human subject should take precedence over the interests of science." That meant that in controlled trials new methods should be tested against the "best current" methods, not some slipshod facsimile of them, even if the best current methods would be no more than a dream to test subjects had they not enrolled in the trial.[1]

But the codes were vague, and at times contradictory, and this particular standard wasn't one that researchers were too keen on. Since doctors didn't universally dole out the best current methods to their patients, circumscribed as they might be by access to resources and information, why should clinical investigators be held to a higher standard? What if subjects didn't mind not getting the best current treatments, and were happy with second-rate—or even third-rate—regimens? What if by offering substandard care in their trials scientists could produce astounding results that might change the face of the world?

It took the disastrous new scourge of AIDS to lay bare the contradictions. When the Centers for Disease Control first reported on a strange immune deficiency in healthy young gay men in 1981, government officials and drugmakers reacted with studied indifference. So hostile was the Reagan administration to the interests of homosexuals that the surgeon general was "flatly forbidden to make *any* public pronouncements about the new disease," according to journalist Laurie Garrett.[2] Drug companies were reluctant to develop drugs for the deadly infection because they felt the "target market would be too small," FDA historian Philip Hilts wrote. "It was said that to develop a drug to treat an illness affecting fewer than 200,000 people would yield too small a profit."[3]

For medical researchers, though, AIDS presented a breathtaking vortex of research questions. By 1984, amid intense competition among medical researchers, scientists had isolated the cause of the disease.[4] The culprit was a retrovirus, an organism that can only survive and replicate by pirating live cells. HIV is an especially ominous intruder: it infects the immune system itself, hijacking the command centers of pathogen fighters called CD4 cells and instructing them to cease all activities save sending out copies of their new viral commander. Thus crippled, the body is dangerously vulnerable to infections. The retrovirus replicates at a rapid clip, churning out ten billion copies every day, some proportion of which have slight variations—mutations—that would make treating the disease complex.[5]

It was several years and thousands of deaths later before a drug that fought the virus appeared on the scene. Articulate, angry, and accomplished activists such as Larry Kramer, an impassioned playwright, were convinced that if they pushed the NIH, the FDA, and the drug companies hard enough, viable AIDS treatments would be found. "Laboratories have drugs that they're not giving us," fumed Kramer in 1995. "I think that they should go before the equivalent of a Nuremberg Tribunal for War Crimes."[6]

Retrovir (AZT), released in 1987 by a company that would later become part of GlaxoSmithKline, wouldn't exactly be the answer to their demands. AZT, a nucleoside analogue, incorporated itself into the RNA of the virus, rendering it ineffective. A sizable public investment had gone into the development of AZT. The compound had been synthesized by government-funded scientists in 1964, the National Cancer Institute had run the tests that revealed its anti-HIV properties, and the government had helped conduct clinical trials on the drug. Nevertheless, the drug's manufacturer decided to charge poorly insured and dying AIDS patients $8,000 for a year's worth of treatment. Aware that it was about to release the only approved drug available for a deadly disease, the company would make AZT its "largest contributor to revenue and earnings," analyst Jonathan Gelles gushed in 1987. "The profit margin will be about three times the company's 13 percent average."[7]

The New York Times, among others, called the price tag "inhuman," and public demonstrations forced the company to moderate its fee, but by 1994, Retrovir was indeed the $1.6 billion company's second bestselling drug, bringing in over $300 million a year.

Lucrative or not, AZT was no cure-all. The drug worked only after being metabolized into its active form, and persisted in the body for just two hours.[8] Half of those who tried it quit soon afterward because of its toxic side effects, such as fatigue and bone marrow problems. Nevertheless, the network of hospitals and researchers organized by the government to coordinate studies of experimental AIDS therapies, the AIDS Clinical Trials Group (ACTG), was recharged with new focus. Perhaps the drug would protect HIV-infected people from neurological damage or from coming down with AIDS altogether. It might even prevent infected pregnant women from passing the virus on to their babies. Soon ACTG researchers would launch massive new trials using the problematic drug. "People were very nervous about having this drug used in thousands of patients so fast," said Maureen Myers, an AIDS researcher with the National Institute of Allergy and Infectious Diseases, but "we also knew we were going to have limited time to do the things we wanted to do."[9] It would be eight years before the drug industry released a new kind of HIV drug.

Throughout those years the public pressure to do something was intense. Already, the ACTG had come under fire for its me- thodical ploddings. "The AIDS Clinical Trials Group has proved to be a massive, dysfunctional failure in its inept efforts to lengthen the lives of HIV-infected people," the activist organization ACT UP charged in 1990. "This skewed application of increasingly lim- ited government research funds must stop immediately," another activist railed in a letter to the *Washington Post*. "We cannot wait."[10]

And yet, few HIV-positive Americans and their physicians were willing to take part in ACTG studies that compared AZT to a placebo, such as one that measured the effects of the drug in re- tarding neurological damage. Even though patients eligible for the trial were not yet sick and would only be involved in the study for a short while, neither patients nor physicians were willing to risk forgoing the newly available AZT, no matter how limited its benefit. After eleven months of recruiting, the study had enrolled only forty out of a needed three hundred subjects. The researchers were forced to drop the placebo group.[11]

Such problems did not plague one of ACTG's most important early trials. In its trial testing whether AZT might prevent preg- nant HIV-positive women from infecting their babies—a trial coded "076"—researchers had happened upon their first real breakthrough. In placebo-controlled trials in the United States and France, AZT had slashed the transmission of HIV from mother to child from 24.9 percent on placebo to just 7.9 percent. In the study 100 mg of AZT had been administered five times a day to infected pregnant women for months before delivery; during delivery, the women got an IV infusion of the drug, and the baby got a dose of AZT syrup every six hours during its first six weeks of life. Given the extensive volumes of drug required, and the med's still costly price tag, the entire regimen cost around $800.[12] As soon as the effect of the drug was clear—the data was ana- lyzed about midway through the trial—the placebo group was dropped and all the mothers were given the AZT regimen, saving one of every seven of their babies from the deadly infection.[13]

It was 1994, thirteen years after AIDS had emerged and ten years after the virus had been isolated, and finally a randomized controlled trial of an HIV prevention method had rendered a positive finding. "There had not been a single randomized trial that proved that *any* intervention for HIV prevention worked. Nothing!" remembers one HIV researcher. "It was a massive opportunity."[14] In a flurry of official action, the CDC announced its recommendation that clinicians offer the therapy to all pregnant HIV-infected women, regardless of their stage of disease or when they showed up at the hospital.[15] Within months the FDA approved the new use of the drug. With a lifesaving intervention available, the Public Health Service announced their recommendation that all pregnant women receive prenatal HIV counseling and testing.[16]

Major breakthroughs followed hard on the heels of 076. At the end of 1995 the FDA approved the first of a new class of anti-HIV drugs, called protease inhibitors, that disable the virus by preventing it from reproducing within immune cells.[17] Less than a year later the first of a third new class of antiretroviral drugs appeared, nonnucleoside reverse transcriptase inhibitors, which block the virus's RNA from converting into DNA, thus preventing it from taking over immune cells.[18]

Bombarding the virus with all three antiretroviral fighters seemed to defang the virus almost entirely. Although pricey—the combination of brand-name drugs could run to $15,000 a year—and complicated, the U.S. news media along with many HIV-positive Americans breathed a collective sigh of relief.

The most pressing questions, it might have seemed, now revolved around how to ensure universal access to the new solutions. But rather than working to overcome the inevitable barriers of poverty and inequity, many AIDS researchers felt compelled to accommodate them. Though combination antiretroviral therapy might turn the deadly disease into a lifelong chronic condition, U.S. officials and researchers alike seemed to believe this was a solution only for HIV-positive people in the moneyed West. Impoverished Africans and Asians might be suffering the brunt of the global burden of AIDS, but in Africa, "they don't have running water and they don't have watches," Hopkins AIDS researcher Tom Quinn said in 2000.[19] Helping ailing Africans gain access to antiretroviral therapies might save lives, according to leading virologist Robert Gallo, but "it will be a tragic mistake if it's not done right." Since Africans "don't know what Western time is," as the director of the U.S. Agency for International Development claimed in 2001, they were unlikely to take their pills on schedule.[20] They might miss a few doses, opening the door for viral mutations that would render the drugs ineffective. "You'll have 'Eureka' and 'Thank you America!' for two or three years—but then you'll get multi-drug resistance," worried Gallo.[21]

Likewise the World Health Organization did not start strategizing about how best to secure sufficient AZT and distribute it to the pregnant HIV-positive women around the world who were passing on the virus to half a million infants every year. With some governments spending as little as $2 a year on health care for each of their citizens, shelling out $800 to save a single baby from HIV struck officials as impossibly expensive. Not only that: according to University of Natal HIV researcher Hoosen Coovadia, the 076 regimen was "scientifically inapplicable to African populations."[22] Most pregnant women in developing countries didn't show up at hospitals in time to start the therapy, typically bearing their babies far from medical clinics where health care workers could administer the IV drugs. And then, even if a baby were saved from infection at birth, the mother was likely to spend months feeding the baby infected milk from her breast.[23]

At a 1994 meeting convened to discuss the 076 breakthrough the WHO decided not to endorse AZT for global use among pregnant women infected with the virus. The regimen had "a number of features (cost and logistical issues, among others) which limit its general applicability," the WHO reported. Nor would WHO devote resources to figuring out how to make 076 work. Instead, "simpler and less costly" therapies for use solely during delivery should be "urgently studied."[24]

The question was: how could researchers conduct ethical experiments in search of solutions that could very well prove less effective than 076?

There is an inherent perversity in controlled clinical trials, which is that by relying on the contrast between two groups treated differently, one group must suffer worse outcomes than the other. In HIV prevention trials that means that one group must suffer more HIV infections than the other. It also means that uninfected people must expose themselves to the virus. Subjects must venture into the ring with the lion, some equipped with armor, the others bare fleshed. It doesn't behoove researchers to hand out shields and swords, though that might save their subjects—then the researchers could never determine whether the armor worked. The more stripped-down the subjects are, the more viciously the lion tears into them, the easier it is for scientists to quickly discern the value of their preventive tools.

A few HIV researchers noticed the potential conflict-of-interest early on in the business of HIV prevention research. Investigators testing new HIV prevention methods would have a built-in incentive to slack off on providing other protective methods to their subjects. When a group of HIV researchers pressed their colleagues in a 1994 paper to ensure that their test subjects were all armed with the best protective measures available, including counseling, free condoms, and sterile needles, the response was tepid at best.[25] "Why would you do that?" a senior scientist grilled one of the authors. "You'd be cutting off your nose to spite your face! Let them get infected! You want to see a difference!"[26]

That paper was written just as HIV vaccine researchers were attempting to circumvent conflict-of-interest problems by siting risky trials in poor countries. By then, the leading HIV vaccine candidate, Genentech's gp120 vaccine, had been roundly condemned as a dud.

The vaccine triggered antibodies, but they had no effect whatsoever on HIV. The immune response the vaccine provoked was nothing like the one seen in the handful of extraordinary people who had been exposed to the virus but somehow had resisted infection. The NIH, which had initially planned to help push the vaccine into large-scale human trials, withdrew its support in June 1994.[27]

Big clinical trials of such a vaccine posed too great a risk to experimental subjects, NIH advisers decided. A dangerously misleading sense of security might fall over those taking an experimental vaccine with the NIH imprimatur. "People will make the assumption that if the NIH and the groups that have come together have felt that we should go ahead, they must really believe that it's going to work," said Anthony Fauci, director of the National Institute of Allergy and Infectious Diseases. Such subjects were at real risk of not taking adequate protective precautions, generally difficult in the first place for the high-risk subjects researchers would need to recruit for the trial. Finally, vaccinees would test positive on HIV tests even if they were not infected, by virtue of having taken the vaccine. This might open them up to discrimination. Some vaccine researchers even worried that the vaccine could make its recipients more susceptible to HIV infection. Genentech started to dismantle its AIDS vaccine program.[28]

Later the same year, however, the World Health Organization met to discuss whether the vaccine trial could, in fact, move forward—in Thailand. Thai government officials needed to "try something," as journalist Jon Cohen put it in his book on AIDS vaccines, *Shots in the Dark*, "even something that had only an outside chance of working." The sexually transmitted infection was decimating their country, including, notably, their commercial sex industry, which was not only their top source of foreign exchange but also almost universally patronized by Thai military recruits. Some critics of the vaccine accused the WHO of being in the pocket of drug companies. "How much did Genentech pay you?" Jean-Paul Levy, then director of France's top AIDS research agency, bellowed at the organizer of the meeting.[29]

In 1995 researcher Don Francis started a new company, Vax-Gen, devoted to developing gp120. With the Thais behind him he didn't need the imprimatur of the NIH. Instead, VaxGen would use $30 million raised from private investors. After all, despite its shoddy showing to date, valuable data might be garnered from subjecting humans to the vaccine, Francis argued. Animal studies were inconclusive at best, and studying how HIV sparred with the vaccine in human bodies could prove useful to developing a better vaccine. VaxGen had already manufactured thousands of doses of experimental vaccine in preparation for a trial.[30] VaxGen would run trials of the vaccine in both the United States and among intravenous drug users in Thailand.

Failing to provide counseling, condoms, or sterile needles—all known to help people avoid getting infected—would hardly be possible in HIV vaccine trials run in the United States. IRBs wouldn't allow it, nor would test subjects put up with it. But elsewhere the situation is different. In 1986, for example, renegade French scientist Daniel Zagury injected an experimental HIV vaccine into healthy children in Zaire even before establishing whether such cells would harm animals, arguing in his defense that conditions in Zaire were so bad that any risk was worth taking if it might save peoples' lives. "You don't know the situation in Zaire," he protested to Cohen. "It's like you're in the desert and you're talking about the level of calcium in the water!"[31] In Thailand VaxGen would not provide their test subjects with the sterile needles that represented their best hope for averting infection. This had nothing to do with the fact that Vax-Gen's financial future depended upon trial results showing that sufficient numbers of control subjects contracted HIV, Francis said. Rather, the company was loath to practice "therapeutic imperialism." Thai officials didn't provide clean needles to drug users, the logic went, so why should VaxGen?[32]

Lanky, affable Jay Brooks Jackson grew up in Ohio, in a family that ran a coal mine. His midwestern roots show in his slow, patient twang, which he punctuates with warm chuckles and folksy "I tell ya's" and "yup's." He earned his MBA in order to work in the family business, but the coal mining life wasn't for him. In his first year on the job union workers staged a long, violent strike. Jackson fled for the sunlit halls of academia.

His earthy pragmatism led him into pathology and chemistry, but then in the late 1980s, the Nobel Prize–winning polio researcher Fred Robbins asked the hardworking, meticulous Jackson to help him set up a new research venture in Uganda, where the AIDS epidemic was burgeoning. In contrast to Jackson's apolitical practicality, the world of AIDS research medicine bristled with fast-talking, ideologically driven activists, scientists, and politicians. But Jackson agreed anyway, and spent the next several years importing computers, generators, and water distillers to establish a state-of-the-art lab at Mulago Hospital in Kampala, Uganda. He knew the esteemed senior scientist who had invited him to Uganda had lofty goals. Robbins wanted to, "you know, help Africa," explained Jackson, awkwardly. But for Jackson it was simply a good job. Humanitarianism "wasn't a conscious thought at the time," he says, laughing and nodding his head. "It was more like, 'Nobel Prize winner? Sure!' "[33]

By 1994, Jackson was a professor of pathology at Case Western Reserve University School of Medicine, and one among many researchers in the ACTG who met to discuss research priorities in the wake of the 076 results. Jackson suspected that a single powerful dose of an immediately active and much longer acting antiretroviral could potentially provide the same effect as the long, complicated regimen with short-acting AZT, at a fraction of the cost. Boehringer Ingelheim made an antiretroviral drug called nevirapine that might do the trick, because it was immediately active and potent for sixty hours with a single dose. At the time nevirapine had essentially fallen off the map in AIDS treatment because of its proclivity for nurturing resistant strains of HIV.

"There were people in ACTG who were talking about using it,"

Jackson recalls. "One guy in particular . . . had mentioned it to me. I remember in the meeting he wanted to do it in Africa. You couldn't do it here [in the United States]! Ethically you couldn't even give AZT for two trimesters and *then* one dose of nevirapine! That was the problem." No American doctor or patient would risk foregoing any part of the now standard 076 regimen, potentially endangering their baby.

But things were different at Mulago Hospital in Kampala, Uganda.[34] Around four thousand HIV-infected pregnant women were delivering their babies at Mulago every year, and of these infants, more than a third would end up with HIV. None of the mothers were able to afford the 076 regimen. If Jackson wanted to test a new therapy out on them, he wouldn't have to pit it against a long course of AZT, since women there would be unlikely to demand it. And he knew he wouldn't be depriving them of something they could get elsewhere. The new intervention, whatever it might be, would be unlikely to work better than 076; Jackson's prediction was that nevirapine might cut the HIV transmission rate down from 25 percent on placebo to 17 percent. But even if it couldn't shake a stick at the 67 percent drop in infections that the 076 regimen could effect, it would be more affordable and so would represent a "highly relevant public health benefit," Jackson contended, and one that was "much more plausible."[35]

Jackson designed a study in which he would administer three different regimens and count how many babies became infected. Around five hundred infected pregnant women would receive a few tablets of AZT during their labor and delivery; another five hundred a single dose of nevirapine. The third group of five hundred women would receive a placebo. Since "the current standard of care [in Uganda] involves no antiretroviral therapy . . . ethically . . . this study will not deny women access to a proven therapy to which they would otherwise have access," he wrote in his proposal to the NIH. None would be encouraged to feed their infants formula rather than infected breast milk, either. "They really can't *not* breastfeed," Jackson said. "The stigma is a huge problem. If you don't breastfeed either you are HIV positive or you don't care about your baby. Two, they don't even have the money to buy the charcoal to heat up the formula let alone buy the formula."[36]

Jackson received a generous grant from the National Institute of Allergy and Infectious Diseases. He'd direct the trial from his new office at Johns Hopkins University in Baltimore, where he'd taken a post as professor of pathology in 1996. Staying on the cutting edge was crucial for Jackson, and it just wasn't possible in Uganda. "You don't have access to journals, and you don't have the meetings and the company, the technology, that you have here," he says, from the vantage point of his spacious, book-lined office, complete with secretaries and hot coffee on request. "Just everything takes longer. Just to send an e-mail takes like ten times longer!" he says, still amazed. "It is slow, it freezes all the time! I mean, you go to work and half the time you get a flat tire! Everything is just . . ." He stops, at a loss for words. Instead, Jackson would pop some malaria-preventing mefloquines and visit the study site for a week or two at a time.[37]

Jackson's trial would be among the largest of the mother-to-child HIV prevention studies going. The CDC planned to conduct placebo-controlled trials, too, testing how a few weeks of AZT given during pregnancy worked in comparison to placebos in hundreds of HIV-positive pregnant women in Côte d'Ivoire and Thailand.[38] The race was on.

No drug companies supported the trials, save by shipping a few free doses to use. By then, the 076 regimen already had slashed the number of American babies born with HIV by over 40 percent.[39]

But just as Jackson prepared to launch his trial, the first inklings of its slippery rationales caught the attention of Peter Lurie, an HIV researcher turned activist whose full-throttle condemnation would later spell the trial's undoing. Lurie, a wiry, bearded man with twinkly blue eyes, grew up in Cape Town, South Africa, nearly abandoning medical school before he realized, during a stint at a health advocacy nongovernmental organization (NGO), that medical research could be used to promote public health. After gaining his MD and a master's degree in public health, Lurie took a plum job at the Center for AIDS Prevention Studies in San Francisco. From there he'd conduct HIV prevention research and use it to make political interventions, for example by producing a seven-hundred-page report that undermined conservative politicians' claims that needle-exchange programs encourages drug use. In 1995, Lurie published a paper describing how World Bank structural adjustment programs undermined developing country economies and could thereby help spread HIV. "It was a very radical argument at the time," he says. "It made a huge ruckus when it came out."

In February 1997, the up-and-coming AIDS researcher flew back to Africa to give a presentation about AIDS and the World Bank to a gathering of African journalists in Abidjan, Côte d'Ivoire. It was a meeting that would change the course of his career.

The meeting was held in French. After giving his talk Lurie settled in to listen to the other speakers. Some scientists from the CDC shuffled to the podium. Lurie was sympathetic to CDC scientists, as the agency had funded his work on needle-exchange programs. The CDC scientists offered a routine description of their ongoing studies on HIV-infected pregnant women. The 076 regimen was too costly, they mentioned, so they were administering "half doses" to the women.

According to Lurie, the audience erupted. Local journalists started yelling. "Who do you think we are?" they shouted. "How dare you give us half doses!"

Lurie stepped to the microphone to pose a question. He didn't think the half doses were such a bad idea—they would certainly be less toxic and more affordable than the full dose, and might work just as well—but wondered what treatment the CDC was comparing this regimen to. The answer: placebos.

"I remember standing there, with my mouth open, and waiting there for maybe fifteen seconds, thinking about it." Meanwhile, he recalls, the journalists at the conference "went insane."

Lurie's mind was reeling. How could the CDC scientists be in equipoise about whether the short AZT regimen—the half dose— was any better than placebo? The long course was remarkably better than placebo, slashing the rate of transmission of the virus from nearly 25 percent to less than 8 percent. Given what researchers understood about how AZT blocked the transmission of the virus, it was logical to assume that a little bit of AZT would be better than nothing at all. If so, how could researchers justify looking these HIV-positive pregnant women in the eye, and allowing them to deliver their babies without any protection?

No, the CDC scientists responded, they really didn't know whether the short course of the 076 regimen would work. In fact, they suspected that the 076 regimen was "scientifically inapplicable" in Africa. Their rationalizations seemed strangely familiar to Lurie.[40]

Just that month Alfre Woodard and Laurence Fishburne had starred in an HBO movie about the Tuskegee Syphilis Study. The film highlighted how the study hinged on a racist presumption of the time: the sense among scientists that there were biological differences between black people and white people.[41] Was this the argument being made about the 076 regimen in Africa? That drugs proven effective for Westerners would somehow not work in black Africans? Only such a presumption, Lurie realized, could explain the researchers' state of confusion over whether the short course of AZT would be any different from placebo. Lurie got up again to try to pose the question, but he never got that far. As soon as the word "Tuskegee" escaped his mouth, the organizer, a French AIDS advocate, announced, "I disagree with that!," ordered Lurie's microphone to be cut off, and instructed the translators to stop translating.[42]

Later, when he got back to the United States, a bit of sleuthing revealed to Lurie that the CDC, the United Nations's Joint Programme on HIV/AIDS, UNAIDS, and others were conducting no fewer than fifteen different trials testing experimental interventions to block mother-to-child HIV infections in developing countries.

All fifteen trials pitted their experimental therapies against placebos, reasoning, as Jay Brooks Jackson had, that placebos were no worse for HIV-infected women in poor countries than what they would normally encounter, that is, no treatment at all. This meant that Western scientists were allowing hundreds of HIV-infected pregnant women in their care to deliver their babies unprotected.

Lurie knew that his colleagues had a fondness for placebo-controlled trials. And such trials certainly had their place, Lurie agreed. But if researchers knew that effective treatments were available, they had a clear ethical obligation to provide them, whether that muddied their data or not. Not only would these trials condemn scores of infants to HIV infection, but the trials would set a dangerous precedent. "With the increasing globalization of trade . . . it is likely that studies in developing countries will increase," he'd later write. In the years ahead drug industry researchers could use the same argument—it's no worse than what they would have received anyway—to dole out second-rate care to test subjects in poor countries, or, indeed, to poor patients in rich countries as well.[43]

Of course the interventions under study were important and urgent. Lurie understood that as well as any HIV prevention researcher did. The question was how to balance the rights of research subjects with the goals of the research. If AIDS researchers were seen as undermining human rights, or exploiting people's poverty, their grand collective aim—saving the world from the virus—would be gravely undermined. And in any case, innovative study designs using sophisticated statistical techniques made it possible to both provide the best care to research subjects and gather relevant data for impoverished societies. A Harvard researcher, Marc Lallemant, was doing just that, testing short courses of AZT against long courses of AZT among HIV-positive pregnant Thai women, an "active-controlled" trial in which all test subjects would be treated with something that might prevent their babies from falling ill. Such a trial might take a bit longer and require more test subjects to render a result, but the risks to the participants was greatly lessened. Surely the others could do the same, Lurie thought.

With the help of the health watchdog group Public Citizen, Lurie held a press conference to publicize his critique. With any luck, bringing the problem to public attention would persuade researchers to redesign their studies, averting hundreds of unnecessary HIV infections in African and Asian babies. Although he often spoke in expletives, Lurie was a man of reason. And the outspoken physician had already taken on powerful foes—the White House, the World Bank—and survived to tell the tale. His critiques of the grand poobahs of AIDS research would be no different, he assumed.

He couldn't have been more mistaken.

In September 1997, the *New England Journal of Medicine* published a paper by Lurie and Public Citizen's Sidney Wolfe, MD, articulating their objections to the trials. In a bold editorial accompanying the paper, editor Marcia Angell applauded Lurie's critique and condemned researchers' justifications that substandard care to research subjects wasn't unethical when it was no worse than what they might have received if left to their own devices. The Declaration of Helsinki couldn't be clearer, she argued: research subjects were owed the best standard of care, not whatever might be locally available. "That reasoning is badly flawed," she wrote. "It seems as if we have not come very far from Tuskegee after all." It was that word again. When the *New York Times* saw it they promptly pasted the controversy on the front page of the paper. Now one of the cardinal rules of the research community—never involve the lay press—had been breached.[44]

The reaction was swift and hostile.

Within weeks members of the *Journal's* editorial board—David Ho and Catherine Wilfert—had resigned in outrage. Johns Hopkins University's Alfred Sommer, dean of the school of public health, publicly announced he was "quite honestly appalled at these people." Angell and the South Africa–born Lurie, he said to the *Baltimore Sun*, were "Americans who have absolutely zero experience, have never been involved in changing scientific paradigms or changing policies. They are getting involved in an issue about which they know nothing."[45] Lurie's boss in San Francisco called to say that Lurie's conduct was unethical and unprofessional, and that he would be making that point to the surgeon general, the head of the NIH, and the head of UNAIDS—the top funders in Lurie's field. Johns Hopkins University's Neal Halsey called the vice president for research at the University of Michigan, where Lurie was temporarily stationed, to press him to open an investigation into Lurie's "unprofessional conduct." Even Lurie's brother, Mark, then a doctoral candidate at Johns Hopkins, suffered from the fallout. One of his thesis advisers, AIDS researcher Andrea Ruff, who spearheaded one of the controversial trials, withdrew from his committee.

In October 1997, the Johns Hopkins department of epidemiology held a "discussion" in which Halsey, Sommer, and others aired their defense to the swirling accusations. The Western standard of care would "never be applicable" in Africa, they insisted. Active-controlled trials would render "uninterpretable results," they said. Lallemant's active-controlled study wasn't just bigger and slower than placebo-controlled trials, they said; it was a "disaster."[46] Meanwhile, thousands were dying every day, not for want of the unaffordable antiretroviral therapies that were saving lives in the West but for lack of the kinds of easier, cheaper interventions that researchers from Hopkins and elsewhere were looking for. Sommer himself had spent years trying to convince developing countries of the benefits of vitamin A supplements on child mortality but had found that no volume of data would persuade government officials save placebo-controlled trial after placebo-controlled trial. Sommer kept at it, continuing to deprive children in his placebo groups the simple vitamin well after he had proven to himself that the vitamin could save their lives. Such was the business of saving lives in the third world, he insisted.

Sommer and company were angry. What really rankled was comparing their well-intentioned trials to the Tuskegee study. "It is really inappropriate and pejorative to compare this to the Tuskegee study," said bioethicist Norman Fost in a National Public Radio program on the controversy. It was "gratuitous and almost insulting," added South African AIDS researcher Jerry Coovadia.[47] It didn't help that the implied accusation hailed from Lurie. "Here was this white South African," University of Virginia bioethicist Jonathan D. Moreno remembers, "saying *we* are racist."[48]

But more important, they were threatened. A whole body of research was in jeopardy. If known effective treatments were always provided to test subjects, researchers would only be able to garner useable data when their experimental drugs and methods were as good or better than the stuff already known to work. It was a dangerous idea, as Halsey and others detailed in a flurry of articles in the medical press. How would researchers ever be able to discover affordable interventions like oral rehydration, or micronutrient supplementation, or low-cost surgical techniques if they had to compare them to the standard of care in the cash-flush, technology-rich West? These techniques were, indeed, less effective than the Western standard of care—but more relevant for saving the lives of people with little access to health facilities and inadequate budgets.[49] "There is a global obligation to diminish the worldwide disparities in health care," leading HIV researchers and bioethicists allowed in a joint 1999 *Lancet* paper. But "to expect this profound global injustice to be rectified soon is unrealistic."[50]

In March 1999, CDC scientists announced results from their placebo-controlled trials. The short course of AZT halved the transmission of HIV, compared to placebo. In Bangkok and Abidjan thousands of HIV-infected pregnant women had jostled for entry into the trials, where the white-coated docs might—or might not—dole out drugs to save their babies from infection. Over three hundred of those who made it into the trials did not receive AZT, but rather sugar pills. Nearly seventy of their babies came into the world infected with HIV.[51]

The top AIDS researchers and bioethicists who defended the studies wrote a bold "consensus statement" that accompanied the CDC results. The statement began by arguing that these kinds of trials were important and necessary, despite breaching the ethical principle of assuring research subjects the best care. They said the ethical principles themselves had been misinterpreted. According to the statement, placebo treatment of people who couldn't afford to buy effective medicines was the de facto best standard of care. Researchers, no matter how richly endowed with NIH grants, owed such patients no more than that. "You don't want to deny treatment to anyone who would otherwise get the treatment," said Sommer. But "you're going into Africa where nobody gets anything because the drug is too expensive."[52]

The statements' authors argued that it was "ethically permissible" to administer placebos to HIV-infected pregnant women in countries where antiretrovirals were unavailable. Researchers should provide only the "highest standard of care practically attainable in the host country," they opined. "There is no obligation to provide study participants with the highest standard of care attainable elsewhere in the world."[53] UNAIDS agreed, in a guidance document released the following year.[54]

As for Lurie, he had found himself out of a job within two months of the publication of his *New England Journal* paper. His employers at the Center for AIDS Prevention Studies held a major international conference on HIV prevention and failed to even invite Lurie to speak. Enraged and hurt, Lurie quit. "I was furious! I felt incredibly betrayed!" he says passionately, years later. According to Lurie, his former boss had spoken to the surgeon general and the head of the NIH about Lurie's activities. He hasn't worked in AIDS prevention research since.[55]

* * *

VaxGen's trials of its gp120 vaccine in five thousand gay men in the United States and twenty-five hundred intravenous drug users in Thailand commenced in 1999. Several AIDS researchers took exception to VaxGen's bypassing the NIH decision by moving forward with the Thais. "Majority scientific opinion," said AIDS researcher John P. Moore, had condemned the gp120 vaccines as failures, but still VaxGen and others "cling to their investments." Furthermore, they had seduced desperate health ministers and scientists from developing countries with false hope, then paraded their newfound supporters at international conferences to back them up. "I despise . . . Don Francis and all the evil corporate politics you stand for," railed Moore. "Trying to make money out of the dying is pretty pathetic, really." VaxGen was "abusing the Thai people for selfish reasons," he said. Aaron Diamond AIDS Research Center's David Ho agreed. During a visit to Bangkok Ho warned, "For me as part of the Asian minority in the U.S., I feel it's important for the Thai people to be aware of the possibility of exploitation. . . . If a product is rejected elsewhere, why should you take it? . . . It's wrong for some U.S., European, and other researchers to look at this only as an opportunity to develop a product."[56]

Providing treatment for the subjects who did become infected in the trial was another sticking point. The VaxGen vaccine was unlikely to protect anyone from an infection, researchers knew, but it might slow the course of the disease. If they treated infected subjects with the lifesaving drugs, it might be difficult to tell if the vaccine had any such effect. Drug treatment could "make . . . it impossible to design a scientifically valid [vaccine] trial," worried one Johns Hopkins vaccine researcher. It would also burden the vaccine trials with huge drug bills. "This is a monstrous responsibility," sputtered another clinician. Wouldn't it be unethical, anyway? If they *did* provide the drugs, then people—as yet uninfected with the virus—might sign up just to get the free treatment.[57]

A compromise solution was found in the design of the trial. In the U.S. arm, for every subject who received a placebo, two would receive the vaccine. They'd also get triple-drug therapy should they become infected with the virus. In Thailand, things would be different. There'd be one placebo given for every active shot. If subjects became infected, they'd get therapies, but not triple-drug therapy, just double-drug therapy. "It works," said Lurie with disgust, "but not too good."[58]

After the CDC's placebo-controlled trials proved that short-course AZT cut HIV transmission nearly as well as the long course, pressure was stepped up on Jackson to drop the placebo group in his trial in Uganda, code-named HIVNET 012, as well. Now that researchers knew beyond a shadow of a doubt that even an affordable short course of AZT—around three weeks worth, given during pregnancy—would help, there could be no decent rationale to withhold the drug from any HIV-infected pregnant woman, CDC advisers told Jackson.

Jackson was aghast. Left with just one group of women taking nevirapine and another taking an even more abbreviated course of AZT—just a couple of pills during labor and delivery—Jackson worried that he might be left with uninterpretable results. "If they had turned out to be similar, we wouldn't have known if neither of them worked or both of them worked," he recalls. Such inconclusive results, while surely suggestive, would be less likely to find their way into a top-tier journal. Journal editors frown upon fuzzy results, and Jackson knew it. "At the time, I tell you, it was like, this is crazy!" he says. "If we drop this placebo, chances are we won't be able to say anything!" He had received a very large grant to look at an interesting question and had jumped through many administrative hoops in order to get his study started. To then not be able to publish any papers would clearly have been disastrous. Plus, his earlier argument, that withholding the best methods was permissible since the women wouldn't have gotten better care anyway, still held, he said in 2003. "They said, well, the short course is effective and everybody should just implement it. Well, here we are six years later and nobody is getting it! And we knew that! People knew afterwards that this was wishful thinking. We knew that the standard of care would still be nothing for years to come."[59]

But in the end, the aborted placebo arm in Jackson's trial didn't disrupt the study. In September 1999, Jackson and his team published results from HIVNET 012. The nevirapine had worked even better than the ultra–short course of AZT they had administered—and was easier and cheaper. Of the placebo babies born before the placebo group was dropped 36 percent contracted HIV, as did 20 percent of the babies who got the ultra-short course of AZT. Of the nevirapine babies, only 7 percent came down with HIV.

The public response was tremendous. In Uganda the results were announced by the Ugandan minister of health; in the United States, Vice President Al Gore did the honors. "It was a big deal, one of the highlights of my career," Jackson remembers. "It was high risk, but it was also high return. For me, it's personally been very satisfying. . . . We struck gold with nevirapine."[60] Within a few years Jackson would single-handedly command one of the biggest medical research budgets available to any investigator in the world: nearly $30 million in federal and private grants for AIDS research.[61]

While Jackson basked in the glory of his results, Lallemant's active-controlled trial was still enrolling patients. Although conceived in 1994, Lallemant's trial didn't commence until 1997. The Harvard researcher had spent over a year convincing skeptical NIH advisers that he didn't need a placebo group.[62]

And now hundreds of thousands of babies could be saved with cheap, easy, single doses of nevirapine. Jackson had a suggestion to make it even easier, which he and his team outlined in a paper accompanying his results. Why not just give a nevirapine pill to *every* pregnant woman in countries where HIV ran rampant? It would be easier and cheaper than testing and counseling each one to figure out which ones had the virus. It wasn't as if the women really wanted to know whether they had the virus or not, since antiretroviral treatment was still prohibitively expensive anyway. This way, even if the mothers dropped dead, clueless as to what killed them, their babies might survive. Critics wondered whether such universal drug dosing would suck up vital foreign exchange in poor countries while dismantling vitally important counseling and testing programs that supported Ugandan families of HIV-positive women—the people who would likely care for the women's orphaned children—in a myriad of other ways. Jackson responded with a popular refrain, which he'd repeat in papers and interviews on the subject: "don't make the best the enemy of the good."[63]

Charity groups quickly started distributing nevirapine in their clinics in poor countries. But strangely, some of the worst-hit countries in the world remained stubbornly resistant to the drug's wonders.

6

South Africa: Drug Trials and AIDS Denialism

Most Americans' lives are so intertwined with the ministrations of Western medicines from childbirth to daily aspirin that belief in its healing prowess is nearly an article of faith. But this isn't so in most of the rest of the world. About 80 percent of people living in developing countries—together comprising 64 percent of the total world population—rely on traditional healers, not Western biomedicine, according to University of California pharmacologist Mannfred Hollinger.[1] And in parts of the world where Western medicine's foothold is flimsy at best, shoddy clinical trials can fuel a corrosive mistrust that undermines allopathic medicine more generally, with potentially devastating results.

Nowhere has this phenomenon been more apparent than in South Africa, where periodic controversies over flimsy subject protections in clinical trials ignited a volatile mix of racial resentments and mistrust accumulated over nearly fifty years of apartheid.

Between 1948 and 1994 the white minority in South Africa, descendants of Dutch, German, and French immigrants, doled out rights and privileges according to a schizoid system of racial apartness, "apartheid" in Afrikaans, the Dutch-like language they originated.[2] When AIDS first emerged in the mid-1980s white conservatives in the country rejoiced openly. "If AIDS stops black population growth," one said, "it would be like Father Christmas."[3]

Apartheid had already started a slow genocide among black Africans in the country. Between 1960 and 1983 South African police had forcibly relocated over three million nonwhite South Africans from their homes into racially segregated "townships" and "homelands," isolating them from the rest of society. While the government devoted 97 percent of its health care budget to high-tech specialized care, culminating in a revolutionary heart transplant in Cape Town's Groote Schur Hospital in 1967,[4] blacks were suffering forty-eight times more typhoid fever than whites and their children were dying from easily preventable diseases such as measles. In the townships tens of thousands of people might share a single water spigot. Conditions such as kwashiorkor, a severe form of malnutrition, raged, but the health department failed to take even minimal control measures. Black patients died waiting for ambulances to pick them up, while those reserved for whites idled nearby; those who survived the wait sometimes perished outside empty white hospitals that refused to let them enter.[5]

Notwithstanding notable exceptions, the mostly white South African medical establishment complied with apartheid's strictures. Some medical researchers openly studied the supposed inferiority of blacks and new bacteria that might selectively injure or kill them. The South African Medical and Dental Council extolled the physician's right to "decide to whom he or she wanted to render a service in non-emergency situations." Doctors worked for the security police, witnessing whippings and other torture, and signed off on fraudulent reports that those who succumbed were victims of accidents or suicides.[6]

When the apartheid regime finally fell to the African National Congress (ANC) in 1994, the problem of AIDS remained off the official agenda. ANC loyalists suspected that racist Western researchers had exaggerated the problem. Back in the 1980s NIH researchers had in fact circulated grossly inflated reports of HIV infections in African countries—Robert Gallo had reported that two-thirds of schoolchildren in Uganda were infected; National Cancer Institute researcher Robert Biggar, that between a quarter and one-half of the Kenyan population hosted the virus[7]—based entirely on faulty assays.[8] Hasty conclusions about HIV originating in Haiti had crippled that impoverished nation's tourism industry.[9]

When Kenyan leader Daniel arap Moi condemned AIDS as

nothing more than some "new form of hate campaign" against African economies,[10] many ANC supporters agreed. "It seemed far-fetched that a disease would conveniently kill fags, prostitutes, drug users *and* blacks," recalls one South African ANC loyalist. "It was a Reaganite wet dream!"[11]

The comforting illusion that AIDS was an overhyped nonproblem wouldn't remain intact for long. By the mid-1990s the virus's rampage on the continent had become all too clear. But the Western AIDS establishment once again appeared unhinged from African realities. Many now proclaimed that Africans were too backward for combination antiretroviral therapy, suggesting a vicious indifference to the plight of impoverished Africans.

The insinuation that Africans couldn't be trusted with antiretroviral drugs outraged South African nationalists such as shaggy-haired activist physician Costa Gazi. Gazi had spent two years in prison during apartheid, and says he feels the same way about the fight against AIDS as he did the struggle to end apartheid. "Diabetics living in rural areas get tested once a month; we don't say let's not treat them!" Gazi says.[12]

When at last in 1997 South African legislators amended the country's Medicines Act to allow the health minister to make HIV medicines affordable by breaking patents and buying cheap generics, Western interests appeared once again committed to blocking Africans from accessing the lifesaving meds. Though the measure only applied during health emergencies or when patented medicines were unaffordable, thirty-nine major drug companies marched into court to prevent the law's implementation. "The law is arbitrary and gives the health minister too many powers," Mirryena Deeb of the trade group Pharmaceutical Research and Manufacturers of America (PhRMA) complained. "The minister can make a decision that a drug is too expensive and the drug companies have no right to defend themselves." The Clinton administration promptly placed South Africa on its "watch list" of patent pirates.[13]

With earlier suspicions about the Western medical establishment thus reinforced, ANC officials set about finding an African solution to the problem. In 1997, Thabo Mbeki, then a prominent ANC official, believed he had found one such solution in a drug called Virodene. Virodene was cheap and, according to its University of Pretoria developers, remarkably effective against AIDS. The South African Press Association accepted the developers' claims as they were presented to President Mandela's cabinet. "South African researchers find a cure for AIDS for fifty rand a month," local headlines blared.[14]

Within days the fact that data supporting Virodene had not undergone standard peer review and stemmed from a single trial involving twelve people emerged, and apartheid's ruling party, the National Party, was calling for the ANC health minister to be sacked for supporting the drug. By April 1998, German researchers established that Virodene was an industrial solvent that caused severe liver damage and had no effectiveness against AIDS.[15] When the mostly white media and white medical establishment lambasted Mbeki for his error, ANC supporters took it as an affront. "If they had their way, we would all die of AIDS," the health minister muttered.[16]

It may not have bothered Mbeki that Virodene had been rejected by drug regulatory officials in the country, because as he would later expound, such officials along with much of the rest of South Africa's medical establishment were still dangerously biased against Africans. The South African Medical and Dental Council had retained most of their senior staff from the years of apartheid. The council hadn't investigated reports of medical negligence, fraud, or human rights violations committed by doctors under apartheid. According to a scathing report by Physicians for Human Rights, the "vast majority" of South African doctors accused of abusing patients during the apartheid era still practiced medicine, in some cases holding top positions in the government, universities, and other institutions.[17]

By the time Mbeki took the helm of the South African government in 1999, his antipathy toward the Western AIDS establishment had gone rigid. According to Mbeki, received truths from

Western AIDS experts were a mix of lies and half truths. The idea, promoted by Western AIDS researchers, that HIV came from Africa was "wild and insulting," he said. They claimed that the disease could only be tamed by expensive, Western-made anti-retroviral drugs, despite what he called a "large volume of scientific literature" that deemed the drugs "a danger to health." In fact, according to Mbeki, HIV was harmless and the condition called AIDS was simply a new name for malnutrition and other diseases of poverty. By then, about one-quarter of all pregnant women in South Africa appeared to be carrying the virus, according to annual antenatal surveys, but the government refused to pick up the tab for any antiretroviral drugs to treat the women or prevent the virus from infecting their infants.[18]

In desperation, physicians like Gazi had taken to smuggling in bags of nevirapine pills from the United States to provide to their pregnant HIV-positive patients. Mining companies such as Anglo-American, realizing that they could lose nearly one-fifth of their miners to the disease, offered to provide antiretroviral combination therapy to their employees. But the overwhelming majority of AIDS sufferers in the country went untreated, and the virus continued its passage from mother to child unimpeded. By 2003, South Africa was home to the greatest number of HIV infected people on earth. Most had never swallowed a single antiretroviral pill, a decade after the approval of AZT and years after combination antiretroviral therapy had transformed the disease in the West.[19]

These demographics did not go unnoticed by drugmakers and CROs casting about for new test subjects to service the $5 billion AIDS-drug market, one projected to mushroom to nearly $15 billion by 2007.[20] CROs flocked to the country to conduct trials on untreated South Africans, and cash-starved medical facilities welcomed them with open arms. At institutions like the University of Stellenbosch drug companies would soon be proposing over sixty new trials every year.[21]

Industry researchers struggled to discern the effect of their new drugs in Western patients who already had dozens of other meds coursing through their veins. "You want relatively clean patients, with no other disease states and no other treatment," explained Simon Yaxley of MDS Pharma, a company that recruits experimental subjects in Eastern Europe, South Africa, Latin America, and China for multinational drug companies. "Then you can say relatively clearly that whatever happens to that patient is from the drug." For testing new AIDS drugs, he said, "South Africa is a great country. . . . There are a lot of individuals [with AIDS] who are not treated."[22] Indeed, echoed a PhRMA spokesperson, "treament-naive patients"—those who have never been exposed to any drug treatments—are "a very important group."[23]

For former Genentech marketing executive Richard Hollis experimental access to South Africa's med-deprived masses would prove crucial. A squat, richly suited man with closely cropped hair, Hollis had left Genentech to "create a new Eden on earth," by selling miracle cures through his new start-up drug company, Hollis-Eden.[24] In 1994, Hollis had acquired rights to a steroidal hormone that he hoped might help prevent the onset of AIDS in HIV-infected people. The trouble was that his scientists could only measure the drug's effects in HIV-infected people if they weren't already taking antiretroviral drugs. Powerful antiretroviral therapy would mask the weak effects of the humble steroid as an espresso would a cup of chamomile tea.

The drug, Immunitin, could nevertheless be worthwhile, Hollis said. "If we're correct in our approach, we could potentially help more than 1 billion people," he proclaimed. After all, "you can't go to third-world countries with $10,000 therapies," he said. "You have to produce drugs that are inexpensive to manufacture and easy to administer."[25]

In 1998, the CRO Quintiles helped the company arrange a short, three-month trial of Immunitin on forty untreated HIV-positive patients in South Africa. According to the disgruntled local press, "the firm want[ed] to avoid the expense of satisfying US regulators until SA guinea pigs have proved that the investment is worthwhile."[26] (Six months later the company did start a trial of the drug in American patients but there the FDA insisted that the company only enroll patients whose antiretroviral drugs had stopped working.[27])

When the results of the 1998 trial turned out to be inconclusive, investors started getting snappish about the company's ability to get a drug on the market. "They may have the greatest thing since chopped liver, but no one is biting," one wrote in 2000. "Investors aren't quite sure what is going on, if anything is going on."[28] The company quickly slapped defamation suits on one of its critical stockholders[29] and launched a longer, more rigorous trial of Immunitin. This time, they'd test Immunitin in much sicker un-treated AIDS patients.[30] Twenty-five South Africans dying of AIDS—their CD4 cell counts numbered less than fifty, well below the two-hundred-count level considered dangerous—were duly enrolled. None were given antiretroviral drugs. Half were given Immunitin in the hope that it would protect them from oppor-tunistic infections. The other half were given a placebo. Hollis-Eden tracked their deterioration for over a year. Eight months into the study, Richard Hollis donned an African-style tunic to have his picture snapped with Nelson Mandela.[31]

Later, data in hand, the company sighed contentedly. "We proved our point," exulted one Hollis-Eden executive. The Immunitin had indeed slowed the deterioration of some of the patients, although the numbers were small. Whatever happened to the test subjects af-ter the one-year trial, the company didn't really know. If they had wanted more Immunitin, they would have been out of luck. The company stopped providing the drug after the study ended.[32]

Finding few Western donors interested in paying for a non-antiretroviral agent for their AIDS programs and governments ca-pable, if they wanted, of overriding the company's patent on Immunitin, in 2002 Hollis-Eden put its Immunitin development program "temporarily on hold," according to its 2004 report to in-vestors.[33]

*   *   *

Meanwhile, other clinical researchers in South Africa, even those conducting more patient-friendly protocols than Immunitin's year-long placebo trial, were getting caught coercing and misinforming their research subjects. "Many patients have no idea what their rights are as patients, even in a therapeutic setting," says University of Stellenbosch bioethicist Keymanthri Moodley. "A lot of people get away with many things in South Africa!"[34]

In 1999, for example, Quintiles had helped a subsidiary of the $11 billion biotech company Gilead launch a five-hundred-patient trial of its new antiretroviral, Emtriva.[35] Some subjects complained about the trial to Costa Gazi who, as the health spokesperson of the dissident Pan Africanist Congress Party, set off to investigate. According to Gazi, one patient was told neither that the drug therapy wasn't a cure nor that he was allowed to leave the study. Others added that the informed consent process consisted of a few minutes' long conversation and an instruction to "sign on the line to get a drug that will cure them." Still others said they were never asked for any written consent at all.[36] As for the ethics "committee," it consisted of a single retired professor.[37]

When patients in the trial started perishing, mistrust between test subjects and investigators surged. After the sixth patient died the researcher in charge of the study site where the death occurred flatly denied the patient had been enrolled, or had even taken any AIDS drugs, despite the fact that reporters had acquired a copy of her consent form inducting her into the trial.[38]

But what had killed the test subjects? They were sick with AIDS, after all. And the regimen given to subjects, unlike in the Immunitin trial, was quite involved. Some were given Emtriva along with d4T and nevirapine; others lamivudine along with d4T and nevirapine.

According to Gilead's consulting scientist, University of the Witwatersrand's Ian Sanne, the liver failures that had contributed to some of the deaths stemmed from the nevirapine, a conclusion Sanne and other Gilead scientists later published in the *Journal of Infectious Diseases*.[39] That is, the same drug that was just then being recommended, thanks to Jackson's 012 study, for South African pregnant women and their newborns. True, in the Emtriva study patients sick with AIDS had taken nevirapine for months on end—to prevent infections in babies, only a single dose was necessary. Prescribed in this way, nevirapine had the potential to save thirty thousand South African babies from HIV infection every year.[40] But to Mbeki such distinctions hardly impinged upon the facts as he saw them: "Our people are being used as guinea pigs and conned into using dangerous and toxic drugs," he insisted.[41] "It would be immoral and unethical for government, despite the numerous requests we are receiving . . . to attempt to make policy decisions regarding the use of nevirapine in our country," Mbeki's health minister declared in 2000.[42]

A few months later nevirapine's manufacturer, Boehringer Ingelheim, announced it would give away the drug for free for use in preventing infant infections in developing countries for a period of five years.[43] But Mbeki's government would not be budged. A year after the Emtriva scandal, and two years after the 012 results established the drug's efficacy, South African regulators reluctantly licensed nevirapine—after countless public articulations of doubt of its efficacy—to prevent mother-to-child transmission of HIV. But the government refused to provide it to clinics and hospitals.[44] Was their expressed dissatisfaction with the drug—it was too dangerous and costly, they said—really the motive? Or was it, as some cynical bystanders wondered, "more a question of: what are they going to do with all of these orphans and how are they going to support them when their parents both die?"[45]

NGOs took the government to court to try to force them to provide the nevirapine. Finally, in March 2002, the health ministry's final appeal failed and the High Court in Pretoria ordered the government to give nevirapine to all HIV-positive pregnant women at public facilities that were capable of doing so.[46]

But new developments in the nevirapine saga would stymie the court's decision even as it was being handed down.

*   *   *

When Jay Brooks Jackson had first set out to study nevirapine's use in preventing HIV infections in newborns in 1997, the drug-maker, Boehringer Ingelheim, had professed little interest. They even charged the researchers for the quantity of drug used in the study. "Many of these companies wanted to stay away from this in the sense that if it works then they are under tremendous pressure to give their drug away," Jackson says. "That was true of Boehringer—they were worried." The company went so far as to write to Jackson informing him that they would not use his data and had no plans to apply for FDA approval for this use of their drug.[47]

But sometime in 2002, for reasons it has never made public, Boehringer reversed itself. The company decided to ask the FDA for approval to market nevirapine as an HIV prevention drug for mother-to-child transmission, using the widely heralded HIVNET 012 trial as proof of the drug's efficacy.

The problem was that that trial had never been conceived to convince FDA officials of anything, but rather as a public-health inquiry. In industry-sponsored trials aimed at FDA approvals drugmakers generally appoint study monitors to help local re-searchers conform to FDA standards twenty-four hours a day. "I mean, when you are sitting out there in Uganda, nobody comes to help you!" Jackson says, laughing. "The FDA likes documenta-tion, other than the trial data. They want hospital records, to ver-ify adverse events. You know, the FDA has seen a lot of scams, so it is perfectly understandable. But you know, Mulago Hospital! They didn't have records!" Jackson and his team were swept into a frenzy of checking and rechecking documentation, and the NIH sent a consultant to Uganda to audit the trial site ahead of a planned visit from the FDA.

The consultant didn't like what he found.

Under FDA regulations subjects must sign a new consent form whenever the trial protocol is changed: the clinicians hadn't done this after they dropped the placebo arm midway through the trial. They also hadn't secured new consent forms from the guardians of surviving infants when the mothers who had initially consented had died. They hadn't reported adverse events as serious if they could be managed without hospitalization, even though the latest FDA rules defines them as serious. On some documents "people who had made a mistake had just crossed it out or whited it out," says Jackson. "The drug was supposed to be kept at room temperature, and it was, but the temperature wasn't monitored. Lots of little things like that." Upon the consultant's alert the FDA canceled its trip, and Boehringer decided to pull its application.

Although nothing in the consultant's findings nor in the NIH review of the trial that followed undermined the overall findings of the 012 study,[48] the South African government greeted the drug's withdrawal from FDA consideration as vindication of all their doubts. "We can't have double standards," said the health minister in August 2003. "We can't have something that's only good for Africa and not good for developed countries."[49] Nevirapine would be deregistered in South Africa, she declared, unless the drugmaker provided new data within a matter of months.[50] If it were deregistered, anyone caught providing the drug to a patient to prevent HIV infection could be thrown into prison for up to ten years.[51]

Outrage over the investigators' apparent carelessness toward the human rights of research subjects—even in trials designed to promote public health—overflowed into a broader rejection of Western AIDS medicines. "It's not just antiretrovirals" that can be used for AIDS, the minister said. "We've got traditional medicines that we know actually avert AIDS-related diseases.... We are busy studying it ... and we are seeing excellent results."[52] One of the most promising such remedies, according to the minister, combined African potatoes, garlic, lemon, and olive oil. "These things are affordable for South Africans," she said, "not like things like antiretrovirals."[53]

By then, the price of antiretroviral drugs, just five years after the advent of combination therapy, had fallen precipitously. In early

2001, generic drug manufacturers in India had produced a triple antiretroviral drug therapy for $1 a day, or 3 percent of the average cost in the United States.[54] Within a few years over three hundred thousand AIDS patients in the developing world—nearly half of all treated AIDS patients in those countries overall—had swallowed the cheap meds.[55] The thirty-nine drug companies that had dragged the South African government into court over the policy it designed to bring down drug prices abandoned their reputation-crushing lawsuit that same year.[56] By August 2003, when a South African drug company started manufacturing generic antiretroviral drugs, the government's resistance had finally crumbled. According to a surprise announcement by health officials at an AIDS conference in Durban, the government would commit to providing antiretrovirals "as a matter of urgency" and supported the use of nevirapine to prevent infections in newborns.[57]

Not only did suspicions about the motives and practices of clinical researchers contribute to delays in AIDS treatment—and to the loss of lives on account of them—but none of the justifications the research establishment had offered earlier to support their lower standards for subjects in poor countries held up in the end.

From Alfred Sommer to Richard Hollis, Western researchers had insisted that the price of AIDS drugs was too high, the drug regimens too complicated, and active-controlled trials too slow. And yet, while they sought affordable but second-rate treatments, the price of antiretroviral therapy had plummeted. Meanwhile, contrary to the assumptions of many Western scientists, studies had revealed that patients in Uganda and Botswana were actually better at taking their antiretroviral drugs than most Americans, and were more honest about it as well.[58]

Finally, the active-controlled trials derided as disastrous had rendered interpretable results in the same amount of time as the placebo trials. Lallemant's active-control trial was published in October 2000. It had taken about two years from start to finish—as had the placebo-controlled trials run by the CDC and Jackson.

The results were perfectly interpretable.

7

Outsourcing to India: The One Billion Body Politic

Over the last five decades a thicket of ethical principles, regulations, and codes has taken root in the United States, governing relations between subjects and investigators as well as patients and clinicians. However uneven or sparse in places, few physicians or scientists involved in human experimentation can avoid navigating it. But the modern hunt for bodies leads drugmakers to places almost entirely shorn of such oversight. Such is the case in India, where a one billion body bounty entices industry investigators.

Ethical transgressions in clinical research in India periodically surface in the nation's loud and exuberant press. For several decades starting in the 1970s, for example, hundreds of thousands of impoverished Indian women received an unapproved drug, some of them unknowingly, that was distributed by American population control advocates.[1] The drug, quinacrine, burns the fallopian tubes, forming scars that sterilize the patient permanently.[2] In the mid-1980s government doctors had herded village women into a trial of an injectable contraceptive that had been withdrawn from the market for its association with tumors in rats over a decade previously. The women "had no idea they were participating in a trial," recalled an activist from Stree Shakti Sanghatana, a Hyderabad-based women's group. If the women had been informed, paramedics in charge of the trial told Stree activists, no one would have volunteered.[3] Between 1991 and 1999 a government-sponsored trial of a leprosy vaccine failed to mention to the rural participants that the trial was double blind and that some would receive a placebo.[4] In the late 1990s a Tuskegee-like government trial was exposed, in which researchers purposely withheld treatment from over eleven hundred mostly illiterate women with precancerous lesions on their cervixes in order to study the inevitable progression of the disease. They didn't inform the patients or ask for their consent, because, they said, such niceties weren't mandatory when the study began.[5] In 2001, a Johns Hopkins researcher was caught testing an experimental cancer drug, which hadn't been proven safe in animals, on over a dozen patients sick with cancer in the state of Kerala. This researcher had failed to secure adequate informed consent as well.[6]

In 2003, yet another scandal broke. Clinicians sponsored by an Indian pharmaceutical company had administered an experimental drug to over four hundred women, telling them it would boost their fertility. But according to the FDA, the drug, letrozole, is an anticancer agent toxic to embryos. Worse, letrozole had yet to be approved for medical use.[7]

None of these transgressions had led to legal protections for research subjects. "In India, there is no law to safeguard the interests of volunteers involved in clinical trials," Arun Bal, president of the Association for Consumers' Action on Safety and Health, told the *Economic Times* in 2004. "Though the Indian Council of Medical Research has laid down guidelines for conducting trials, there is no mechanism in place to ensure that they are being implemented."[8]

It isn't just clinical experimentation that departed from basic ethics, but clinical practice itself. While a labyrinth of ethical, moral, and spiritual conventions governs nearly every aspect of social life in India, from eating to sex to relationships, government regulation of industry and trade remains thin, and medicine is no exception.

The 1990s had seen a massive boom in new medical schools run by private companies and religious groups. Scandals regularly emerged about the new institutions, which critics likened to certificate-churning money machines. Some had been caught selling admission, others even auctioned medical degrees. Medical schools had been caught temporarily hiring fake teachers to fool inspectors that they had sufficient teaching staff. In 2003, there wasn't a single medical school in the country that taught a course on medical ethics.[9]

Once physicians garner a license to practice medicine, the government does little to ensure that they demonstrate any ongoing competence.[10] Not surprisingly, quackery is widespread. One mid-1990s survey in Mumbai cited in the *British Medical Journal* found "clinics operating out of residential flats, with kitchens turned into operating theaters." Naïve, illiterate patients—as of 2001, 44 percent of the nation's people could not read or write[11]—keep lining up for these informal clinics regardless, as the waits are still shorter than at the woefully underequipped public clinics.[12]

Neither the state medical councils nor the Indian Medical Association take it upon themselves to police physicians' conduct. The Indian Medical Association espouses no code of ethics for its members and has fought off any imposition of minimum standards, whether regarding patient care or licensing. In 1994, when the city of Surat in the northern state of Gujarat suffered an outbreak of plague, three-quarters of the city's physicians promptly fled. State and national medical authorities said nothing about their negligence.[13]

In the late 1980s a small group of progressive physicians hoping to strengthen patient rights and regulatory oversight of medical practice launched an effort to revive the moribund state medical council, running nine ambitious new candidates for positions. But other nominees, intent on the prestige of a council position, had hired goons to collect blank ballots from doctors who, for one reason or another, decided not to vote. They inked their own names on the ballots and submitted them to the council. On the final day of the vote the council offices were crammed with hired hands dropping off sacks of ballots for their bosses. The slate of progressive physicians lost. In the ensuing scandal, the council was disbanded.[14]

But perhaps the most chaotic, unregulated aspect of Indian medicine is its vast market in pharmaceuticals. Since a 1972 law had allowed companies to manufacture patented, brand-name compounds so long as they altered the manufacturing process slightly, a flourishing pharmaceutical industry had sprung up. In 2004, there were over twenty thousand licensed drug companies in the country, including most of the major multinational outfits,[15] flooding the market with over seventy thousand different brands of medicines.[16] (According to the World Health Organization less than three hundred drugs are necessary to control 95 percent of the country's health problems.[17]) To regulate this bewildering array of products the government employs just six hundred drug inspectors.[18]

The illicit marketing of drugs is widespread. In a 2003 raid in Patna, in the eastern state of Bihar, seven out of nine drugstores were found to be operating without licenses.[19] Pharmacists routinely sell prescription-only preparations to patients without a prescription, encouraged by drug giants like GlaxoSmithKline, who shower pharmacists with lavish gifts, including free color televisions, for placing large orders.[20] Drugs are often repackaged into slick combination pills that make little clinical sense, pharmacologists say. Over seventy combinations are not just ineffective but dangerous, and are sold under more than one thousand different brand names.[21] Other drugs are sold for catch-all conditions including "intellectual decay," "social maladjustment," and "deterioration in behavior." Legitimately useful drugs are often sold without any mention of their known adverse effects. According to a 2003 magazine exposé, no less than one in four drugs available on the market is fake or substandard: ground up chalk, sugar, and contaminated tap water masquerading as lifesaving medicines.[22]

But according to Indian industry analyst Chandra Gulhati, MD, "even if an erring company is caught red-handed indulging in illegal activities, it is let off, for reasons best known to regulators, with a light warning."[23]

Rather than reinforce the sagging regulatory gates, starting in the late 1980s, the government opted to introduce yet another element to the anarchic mix: Western-style, for-profit medical services.

During the 1990s Indian leaders shed the nationalistic rules that had protected the nation's medical market from foreign interests and made way for deep-pocketed investors to march in.

By 2002 it was clear to Indian public health workers that "the provision of medical services" in the country had become "big business."[24] Predictably, the new corporate hospitals did not pick up the slack from overcrowded public ones catering to the 4.5 million Indians infected with HIV—the second-largest population of such patients in the world—the millions of Indians suffering from tuberculosis and chronic hepatitis, or the masses of children dying of diarrhea, measles, pneumonia, and even polio.[25] Instead, they sought out elite and upper-middle-class Indians, as well as medical tourists from the UK and the Middle East, providing high-tech specialized care in a business that analysts said could be worth up to $2 billion a year.[26]

Trailing close behind the new corporate hospitals were the multinational drug companies that would stock their formularies. Anticipating a market for drugs that could reach nearly $10 billion within a few years, Pfizer, Chiron, Merck, and GlaxoSmithKline all announced plans to expand their operations in India between 2000 and 2005. Novartis built a gleaming, marble-white building amid the smog-clogged ruins of Mumbai's inner city, and ringed it with expansive emerald lawns meticulously groomed by rail-thin locals. Eli Lilly announced plans to triple its R&D in the country.[27] Once new patent laws required by the WTO muted the generic drug industry, the multinationals' market share would balloon from just a quarter to nearly half by 2010, the *Daily International Pharma Alert*, a trade publication, predicted in January 2005.[28] It didn't bode well for the poor majority. In 2004, Novartis execs had admitted to the World Bank that they viewed India as a market of just 50 million people—that is, the company had no plans to even try to sell its drugs to the other 95 percent of the Indian population.[29]

Government officials hoped likewise to expand the scale of industry-sponsored clinical trials in the country, from a $70 million business to a $1 billion one. During the early 2000s, they eased the way with a series of exemptions and incentives. Experimental drugs would be exempted from customs duties.[30] Companies would no longer have to complete Phase 3 trials in other countries before launching such trials in India. They wouldn't have to demonstrate their experimental drug's "special value" to India anymore either. Companies willing to invest in R&D in India would be congratulated with ten-year tax concessions. In 2003, when the director of an American company that tracks the clinical trials business came to India for a conference, government officials feted him as if he were a head of state.[31]

Over a dozen full-service Western CROs set up shop in the country, all with ambitious plans to expand.[32] "The opportunities are huge, the multinationals are eager, the Indian companies are willing," the *Economic Times* enthused in 2004. "We have the skills, we have the people and we have an advantage which China doesn't and probably never will. Best of all, this is one sort of outsourcing which American workers aren't likely to protest."[33]

But would the country's threadbare ethics infrastructure be up to the task? While in theory clinical sites that conduct trials have to engage the oversight of an ethics committee, in practice such committees are few and far between. Many of those that do meet regularly do so "in order to enable clearance" of proposed trials, not to question their ethics or relevance, Indian health activist Sandhya Srinivasan says.[34] "They hardly meet," agrees Amar Jesani, MD, a Mumbai-based bioethicist who sits on several such committees. "The chairperson will just keep signing. They don't know how to review a proposal from an ethics point of view," he says. "To do work as an ethics consultant in India, you must make more and more enemies. . . . There is no ethics culture in the profession."

Jesani, as one of the founders of the nation's only medical ethics journal, is one of the most prominent medical ethicists in the country. "I'm not trained in ethics at all," he says, leaning back in his chair and chuckling. "I have no degree! When I did medicine, there was no class in ethics!" he declares gleefully. "So nobody is trained in ethics, and I am in demand."

Western drug company executives insist that they can make up for the ethical vacuum. "All global companies follow global protocols when they conduct clinical trials," Ranjit Shahani, MD, vice chair of Novartis India told *Economic Times* reporters in 2004.[35] True, many of the clinicians in India who might be leading the new trials lack training in good clinical practices, but "this may not necessarily be considered negative," said Chandrashekhar Potkar, Pfizer's director of clinical studies in India in 2003.[36] Their training could be entirely directed by drug companies.

Plus, the industry funding on offer for trials could provide improbable medical luxuries amid the general scarcity, as the endocrinologist Nadeem Rais knew well. Rais has been conducting clinical trials for major drug companies at his posh south Mumbai clinic, the Chowpatty Medical Centre (CMC), for years. At public clinics examining rooms might come equipped with a metal desk, a few chairs, a dirty ceiling fan, and ragged pieces of paper pinned under a rock for prescriptions.[37] At the Chowpatty Medical Centre, patients lounge on plush blue couches while waiters, their uniformed lapels emblazoned with "CMC," stride by briskly, ferrying trays of lime soda into the consulting rooms. Rais's air-conditioned office is equipped with two heavy and glistening wooden desks, upholstered seating, and flat-screen computer monitors.

Rais has enrolled thousands of local patients in trials on erectile dysfunction, diabetes, and other conditions for Eli Lilly, Glaxo-SmithKline, and others. "We are always overbooked for trials," he says proudly. On the CenterWatch Web site, which promotes clinical sites around the world for industry trials, Rais boasts that he maintains 90 percent patient "compliance" with trial protocols. "We have electronic medical forms for each patient for the last ten years. We can get any info we want. What do you want to know?" He asks amiably, tossing me one of his patient's medical records. It neatly lists the patient's name, address, and medical history: a middle-aged woman with diabetes, as it turns out.[38]

One subject of a trial at the center, a worker in a shoe store, recalls being "rather awed" by Rais's clinic. The CMC doctors offered him four different cell phone numbers to call upon, free insulin, and four thousand rupees a month, in exchange for a signature on an informed consent form. "Look, I didn't have a stable job; insulin costs 1700 rupees a month. I have two daughters. And I weighed 49 kg [108 pounds]." He joined the trial.[39]

Rais says he doesn't seek to enroll solely poor and working-class patients, but the fact is that middle-class and wealthy Indians are less interested in participating in the kinds of randomized controlled trials that drug companies looking for FDA approval favor. Less than 1 percent of Indians own health insurance, so most pay upfront for their care, scraping together funds from relatives and friends as necessary to do it.[40] While Western hospital wards are studded with Indian physicians, in India itself doctors are at a premium. There is one for every two thousand people.[41] Why would well-off Indian patients, accustomed to arranging everything from shoe purchases to marriages through well-oiled personal connections, willingly substitute their own precious doctor's judgment with that of some randomizing computer?[42]

Because of Indians' strong preference for personal connections, only those who "have absolutely no choice" can be expected to agree to the impersonal care doled out in a randomized clinical trial, says clinical researcher Farhad Kapadia of Mumbai's Hinduja Hospital. And these mostly poor patients who serve as subjects live in a world apart from the socially powerful doctors who experiment upon them.

A 2003 story in a glossy national magazine featured a typical story of the misunderstandings that can result. A woman's uterus had been removed after the delivery of her first child. According to the doctor, the patient was hemorrhaging after the delivery, so the uterus had to be removed to save her life. The patient's story was that the delivery had been botched and her uterus removed to destroy the evidence.[43] Whether the doctor had failed utterly to secure informed consent from her patient, or whether the doctor was a dangerous fraud, or whether the patient's account was un-true, was left unexplained. After another such incident, the death of a patient during minor surgery, an angry mob burned down a hospital in Kerala. There is a "tremendous mismatch between pa-tient expectations and services offered by us," noted the Indian Medical Association's president, Arul Raj.[44]

Given all this, the potential for abuse of research subjects in India appears nearly unlimited. But if in the past government officials tolerated ethical lapses because most experimentation was ori-ented toward public health goals, no such trade-off exists today, for the modern body hunt in India proceeds by the logic not of public health but the profit-driven needs of distant drug companies.

In 2003, Kapadia conducted a trial on behalf of Eli Lilly at Mumbai's Hinduja Hospital, a large, modern facility in the mid-dle of the steaming city. It was the first "proper randomized trial" he had been involved in, and the ambitious young doctor was enthusiastic about participating in the international study. But his patients "are very reluctant," Kapadia said. "I've had more turn-downs than consents." Hinduja Hospital is not luxuri-ous by any stretch of the imagination, but it is clean, well lit, and spacious. The elevators work. There are guards at the front en-trances. The urban Indians who come to this hospital have high expectations. The problem, Kapadia said, lies in the uncomfort-ably frank consent form required by the FDA. It didn't pussyfoot around the risks of the drug or the trial. "It is pretty explicit," Ka-padia said. The drug that Kapadia was testing, Xigris, was not a benign one, nor was the method in which Eli Lilly wanted him to use it.

If Kapadia's research subjects would suffer the consequences, this had less to do with medical necessity or the lack of safer al-ternatives than with competitive pressures in a pharmaceutical market across the ocean in the United States. Eli Lilly had a lot at stake with its latest trial on Xigris. The success of the drug was "central" to the company's "medium-term performance," the *Financial Times* noted in 2002. Lilly's blockbuster drug Prozac had fallen off patent in 2001 and Lilly needed to make up for the lost sales income. If Lilly could prove Xigris safe and effective for use in patients with sepsis, analysts said, the drug could bring in up to $2 billion a year for the company.[45]

Sepsis felled hundreds of thousands of Americans ever year,[46] including 70 percent of those who died in intensive care units.[47] It is a mysterious ailment in which the normal inflammation that comes in response to a bout of infection fails to subside.[48] The consequences can be dire. Blood coagulates into vessel-blocking clots. Fever, shakes, and vomiting may follow. The organs may fail. (When it gets this bad clinicians call the condition "severe sepsis."[49]) One-third with severe cases die within a month.[50] Worse, nobody knows for sure why sepsis occurs, or can predict who might fall prey. With the medical establishment shelling out $17 billion every year treating septic patients, interest in developing new treatments runs high.[51]

But it isn't easy. In the early 1990s the biotech company Centocor had attempted to launch a sepsis drug called Centoxin. The drug, a genetically engineered version of a human protein thought to be deficient in patients with sepsis, had protected animals from septic shock in some early lab testing, but follow-up studies had failed to replicate the promising results. Centoxin's performance in the 543 septic patients in the company's first major human trial was lackluster: as many patients died on the drug as did on placebo. But with $200 million already invested in Centoxin, the company was loath to let go.[52] In a 1991 *New England Journal of Medicine* paper the company re-analyzed its data, separating the gray results into their black and white components. While overall death rates hadn't changed in the drug and placebo groups, in certain sepsis patients—those with pathogenic bacteria in their blood, a condition known as gram-negative bacteremia—the death rates between the group on the drug and the group on placebo had indeed diverged, from 49 percent on placebo to 30 percent with the aid of the drug, the company explained.[53]

USA Today enthused that Centoxin could save tens of thousands of patients every year. "The impact of this is like . . . introducing a drug like penicillin," the paper quoted one awestruck physician.[54] Centocor stock soared to nearly $60 a share.[55] But if some patients had improved on the drug while overall the fate of the entire group of patients hadn't changed compared to placebo, critics pointed out, then clearly some patients—those who didn't have gram-negative bacteremia—had been actively killed by the med. Figuring out which patients would benefit and which might be harmed wasn't straightforward. The tests that confirmed a case of gram-negative bacteremia could take up to forty-eight hours.[56] If docs felt pressured to administer Centoxin before they could figure out whether a patient might benefit from it, sepsis patients who did not have gram-negative bacteremia might start dropping like flies.[57]

When the FDA found other anomalies in Centocor's data, they ordered the company to start a new trial. In the new trial the benefits seen in the earlier one vanished: death rates among patients with gram-negative bacteremia were no different in the drug group than among those on placebo.[58] What's more, over three hundred subjects given the drug died, twenty-eight more deaths than would have been expected had they been given no drug at all.[59] Stock fell to less than $7 a share and the company laid plans to dump its aging stockpile of Centoxin.[60]

With Centoxin's high-profile crash and burn—the *New York Times* ran a lengthy front-page story on the drug's spectacular failure in 1993[61]—Eli Lilly would face a skeptical medical elite with its sepsis contender, Xigris. Like Centoxin, Xigris was a biotech version of a naturally occurring molecule, activated protein C, also thought to be deficient in patients with sepsis.[62] Like Centocor, Lilly planned to charge an arm and a leg for its drug—$7,000 for a single course of Xigris. After all, unlike most areas of medicine, critical-care medicine hadn't been subjected to cost-cutting pressures. "The feeling has always been that if you're sick enough to be in the ICU, you're sick enough to let the doctors do what they need to do," Brown University critical care specialist Nicholas Ward said. "In critical-care medicine, we've pretty much had a Gold Card to do what we want."[63]

Such carte blanche wouldn't have held had a cheap, effective therapy been available, of course. And a slow trickle of papers had appeared over the course of the 1990s showing that, at least anecdotally, low doses of corticosteroids were highly effective for sepsis. Corticosteroids were old drugs with well-understood properties, and a course of generics might run to about $50 or so.[64] But when steroid researchers approached various drug companies to sponsor large-scale controlled trials to prove the drug's efficacy beyond a shadow of a doubt, they were roundly rebuffed. Patents on steroids had long expired and so the drugs were widely available for a pittance. No jackpot of extra sales income awaited anyone who proved how such drugs worked or whether they saved lives.[65]

Xigris, on the other hand, had one of the world's biggest drug companies behind it, and Lilly wouldn't cut corners. In the company's first trial of the drug, known as the PROWESS trial (Recombinant Human Activated Protein C Worldwide Evaluation in Severe Sepsis), they roped in nearly 1,700 patients at 164 centers in eleven countries for a massive placebo-controlled trial.[66] In contrast, the first placebo-controlled study of steroid therapy had enrolled just thirty-one patients.[67] The results were impressive—low-dose steroids had saved sixteen septic patients, while more than half of those given placebos had perished—but even wowed critical care experts had to admit that the trial was minuscule. The lead researcher for the PROWESS trial was Vanderbilt University's Gordon Bernard, MD, a researcher who had debunked high doses of steroids as a treatment for sepsis in 1987. Bernard had precious little truck for its low-dose cousin regimen, calling research supporting it weak and the investigator who led it stupid at a conference in Chicago.[68]

By June 2000, not even two years into the PROWESS trial, Xigris had proven so effective that the experiment was summarily discontinued. It would have been "unethical" to continue enrolling placebo patients, Lilly officials said, and deny them the lifesaving properties of Xigris. The drug had dropped the mortality rate by six percentage points, from 30 percent on placebo to 24.1 percent on the drug. The company analyzed the data every which way and yet the positive outcomes persisted. The effect was "consistent" across all the various subgroups of patients, whether they were only mildly ill or on death's door, elderly or youthful. The main adverse effect was serious—sometimes fatal hemorrhaging—but occurring in just 3.5 percent of patients, neatly balanced by the drug's benefits.[69]

Eight months later the results appeared in an early release edition of the *New England Journal of Medicine,* a privilege reserved for papers with urgent public health implications.[70] The rapid notice wouldn't have made much difference to public health—the FDA hadn't even approved the drug yet so it wasn't available to physicians—but it was key to Lilly's efforts to build a buzz about the drug before it hit the market. The same month that the paper appeared the company arranged for Bernard to cohost a thirty-minute Fox cable television special explaining the dangers of sepsis.[71] Lilly enlisted leading sepsis experts to start spreading the word about Xigris.[72]

But when the FDA analyzed the PROWESS data, they found that Xigris hadn't worked for all patients with severe sepsis all the time, as the company's *New England Journal* paper had said. It had only worked for half the patients—those who were most sick—and even for them it had worked only *after* the company revised the protocol midway through the study.

In the trial, in order to ensure that the septic patients who received the drug were roughly similar in age, severity of disease, and other indicators compared to those who received the placebo, Lilly had evaluated them according to a scoring system, the Acute Physiology and Chronic Health Evaluation, or APACHE II. The scoring system runs from 0 to 71, with higher scores signifying greater likelihood of death. When the FDA looked closely at the results it found that patients' APACHE II scores correlated with their responsiveness to Xigris. For the sickest patients, those with APACHE II scores over 25, the death rate on Xigris had dropped by 12 percent compared to placebo. But for those with scores between 20 and 24 the drug had dropped the death rate by only 4 percent. For patients given Xigris who had APACHE scores under 20, the drug had actually *increased* the death rate by 3 percent. Worse, these patients suffered from the drug's side effects—dangerous hemorrhaging—at the same rate.[73] The company had also altered the trial protocol midway through the experiment; in the first half Xigris had shown no efficacy whatsoever. Xigris only started to work after Lilly restricted the study to "better quality patients," as a Lilly researcher explained to a dumbfounded FDA advisory committee.[74]

The committee was split, ten in favor and ten against, but the FDA approved Xigris in November 2001 anyway.[75] The agency added a single caveat: until Lilly provided more data on how the drug worked for patients with low APACHE II scores, the drug's use would be restricted to patients with APACHE scores over 25. It was a restriction doomed to fail, since the scoring system itself was a "moving window," as a Lilly researcher admitted. If the patient qualified in the morning, could the drug be given in the afternoon? Who knew? Lilly would be banned from promoting any "off-label" uses, but doctors would be free to use Xigris, as with any other approved drug, however they saw fit. Although ignoring the restrictions could result in "very serious consequences for the patient," as one FDA adviser acknowledged, many clinicians might sensibly decide to do just that. Besides posting a lengthy transcript of the advisory committee meeting on an obscure section of its Web site, the agency never publicly rebutted the company's rosy *New England Journal of Medicine* paper touting Xigris's efficacy for all sepsis patients.[76]

With the FDA stamp of approval, the marketing of the drug began in earnest. "New hope for taming deadly shock," ran the *New York Times* headline on a long, approving article, featuring quotes from a single sepsis expert—Gordon Bernard.[77] Lilly dispatched over two hundred critical care specialists, at $1,000 a pop, to deliver promotional lectures about the new drug. It splurged on a special George Benson concert for docs likely to prescribe the drug.[78] In an especially lucrative coup, the company convinced the Centers for Medicare and Medicaid to cover their patients' hefty Xigris bills.[79]

In September 2002, alarmed by the FDA's silence on the potential dangers of Xigris and Lilly's glowing marketing material on the drug, a clutch of critical care experts who had participated in the advisory committee meeting went public with their concerns in the *New England Journal of Medicine*. "We believe there is not sufficient evidence at present for it [Xigris] to become standard of care," Massachusetts General Hospital's H. Shaw Warren, the National Institutes of Health's Anthony Suffredini and Peter Q. Eichacker, and University of Texas's Robert S. Munford wrote.[80]

Sales of the drug flagged. In order to realize the full sales potential of Xigris, the company would have to overcome the confusing restrictions the FDA had affixed to the label, industry analysts commented. But proving the drug worked in less sick patients could be "impractical and expensive beyond belief," one sepsis expert said.[81] To prove any shred of efficacy, more subjects taking the drug would have to be shown to survive than those taking placebos, but if the FDA analysis of the PROWESS trial were borne out, it was unlikely that there would be much of a contrast between their fates. To show a difference, either huge numbers of patients would have to be enrolled or the trial would have to be conducted in places where such patients generally died faster and more frequently anyway. Then again, if the PROWESS trial results were borne out, the drug could actively kill such patients. Those most vulnerable were those who were the least sick to begin with, to boot. They had the best chances of survival without treatment.

Lilly, like other big drug companies, had decided to use India as a major center for its clinical trials in 2002.[82] And so the company looked to India to provide a significant number of subjects for its trial testing Xigris against placebo in sepsis patients with APACHE scores under 25, called the ADDRESS trial (Administration of Drotrecogin Alfa [Activated] in Early Severe Sepsis).[83] In India the potential dangers of the drug for less ill patients weren't widely known, and in 2003 Lilly had even applied to the Indian drug controller's office, unsuccessfully, for permission to sell the drug for all patients with sepsis, not just those with high APACHE scores. As far as investigators like Kapadia were concerned, the main problem with Xigris wasn't its safety profile in less sick sepsis patients, but its cost. Kapadia had read the September 2002 critique of the PROWESS trial in the *New England Journal of Medicine*, but the controversy, according to him, revolved "around the price rather than the drug."[84] In the ADDRESS trial, the drug would be offered for free, a particularly appealing option given that it otherwise cost Indians between 600,000 and 1,000,000 rupees (U.S. $13,000 to $21,000) for a course. Poor Indians had been known to forego lifesaving surgeries on their children for a fraction of that price.[85]

For Lilly, the important thing wasn't the number of patients that developing country sites such as India might be able to induct into the trial per se. (Along with the eleven North American and Western European countries that had provided subjects for the PROWESS trial, Lilly would enlist ADDRESS subjects from a range of developing countries, including Argentina, Brazil, Chile, Croatia, Egypt, India, Lebanon, Mexico, the Philippines, Romania, Russia, Saudi Arabia, Singapore, Slovak Republic, Slovenia, South Africa, and Thailand.[86]) As CROs knew all too well, involving developing countries sped up trials not only because of the ease of rapid recruitment but because their patients provided quick, plentiful clinical "events." As CRO exec John Wurzlemann plainly noted, "If you don't have events, you're never going to finish your trial."[87] In the ADDRESS trial, the main event researchers would be counting was death within twenty-eight days. Sufficient quantities of patients would have to perish on placebo in order to demonstrate that Xigris had an effect of some kind. With overall mortality rates for sepsis patients in developing countries running 60 percent higher than those in the United States, even a relative handful of patients could beef up the death count, increasing the odds of speedy, conclusive results.[88]

While the ADDRESS trial moved ahead Lilly continued its aggressive promotion of Xigris. In March 2004, sepsis experts sponsored by Lilly issued guidelines on the proper treatment of the condition in a prominent journal, *Critical Care Medicine*. Each intervention that might occur to a clinician faced with a septic patient was assigned a grade, with the highest marks awarded to those with the most evidence from the kind of large, multimillion-dollar randomized trials that few other than drug companies can afford. Xigris, not surprisingly, won top marks. Other therapies, including antibiotics and steroids, which were supported by years of widespread use and several independent studies, fared poorly under the grading system because they lacked data from large-scale trials.[89] A dozen professional societies signed on to the guidelines, and the PR firm hired by Lilly organized publicity, distributing the guidelines on free posters, pocket guides, and PowerPoint slides.[90]

That month, a prominent steroid researcher approached Lilly with a proposal for a head-to-head trial pitting Xigris against steroids, a study that could help clinicians finally settle the question as to the relative value of the two therapies. Lilly flatly refused to cooperate. The Xigris marketing was having its effect. Researchers in the field chimed in that such a trial would be unethical, since some patients would be deprived of Xigris.[91]

A few months later steroid researchers strengthened the evidence in favor of that therapy with a meta analysis of all the available data on the drug. According to their *British Medical Journal* paper, safe, inexpensive steroid therapy had been found to be just as effective as a $7,000 course of Xigris.[92]

Lilly ignored the results. At its special three-day conference in Hyderabad, India, in July 2004, hosted for Asian critical care specialists, a Lilly exec extolled Xigris as "the only drug available" to treat patients with sepsis.[93] Xigris's momentum burying steroid therapy appeared unstoppable. In September 2004, online medical experts could be found urging clinicians to use Xigris on all patients with severe sepsis. "Should [Xigris] be restricted to patients with severe sepsis with an APACHE II score >25?" the WebMD Web site asked its critical care expert. "I believe the answer is no," came the prominently posted response.[94]

Lilly scientists repeatedly re-analyzed the PROWESS data, dreaming up innovative new angles from which to present the positive data again and again. It was cheaper to use it earlier rather than later, Lilly scientists found. It worked even better when used with patients with low protein C levels, they discovered. It even worked with patients who weighed over 300 pounds. Lilly dispatched its scientists to professional meetings to trumpet the news.

At one such gathering in Seattle in October 2004, amid a flurry of Lilly presentations underlining the benefits and cost-effectiveness of Xigris gleaned from re-analyses of the PROWESS trial data, a little noticed session quietly ran its course. There was no written abstract for the paper that Edward Abraham, MD, presented that day, as the session was a late-breaking one. It wouldn't appear on the society's Web site later on, nor did it attract the attention of the various medical publishing outfits, reporters, and industry analysts trolling for material at the conference. They were drawn instead like flies to honey to a different late-breaking session that showed that Viagra might work for pulmonary hypertension.[95]

To the select few who gathered that day in the misty city Abraham announced that the ADDRESS trial had been terminated eight months before, over a year early. Of the patients who had received placebos, Abraham said, 17 percent had died. Of the group that had received the drug, 18.5 percent had died. There was worse news, too: in patients who had had recent surgery, Xigris had provoked a 20.4 percent death rate, as opposed to just

16.4 percent on placebo. There hadn't been many patients who had high APACHE scores in the trial—just 321 out of 2,613 enrolled subjects. But even among them, 29.5 percent died on the drug, while just 24.7 died on placebo.

India had been the fifth largest contributor of subjects for the trial, after the United States, Germany, France, and Canada. The subjects from developing countries had suffered the highest death rates overall—nearly double that of subjects from North America and Europe.[96]

In the twelve months following the close of the trial, Lilly did little to publicize the failed ADDRESS trial. The company presented the data only in Seattle and at one other meeting that fall, in Europe. Upon request by the Canadian health authorities, Lilly sent a letter to Canadian hospital administrators, informing them about the trial.[97] Buried in the fine print on the Xigris.com Web site, a small chart appeared mentioning a subset of the data.[98]

When the results finally appeared in the *New England Journal of Medicine* in September 2005, the ADDRESS investigators chalked up Xigris's poor showing to the inexperience of many of the local researchers they had had to rely on. "Many of these centers and countries had not previously participated in critical care trials," they wrote, which "may have affected the patient population included in this study, making it difficult to compare the results of this clinical trial directly with those of other studies . . . such as PROWESS."[99] Nevertheless, word spread in the United States that Xigris was a finicky drug with restricted utility, and by 2004 sales of Xigris amounted to a lackluster $200 million.[100]

In the developing countries that ran the ADDRESS trial, as many subjects perished on placebo as on Xigris. On this basis, one could argue that the trial neither helped nor harmed them. But this outcome wasn't predictable; on the contrary, before the trial started, the evidence suggested that patients would, in fact, suffer from the drug. That the FDA and the company moved forward regardless illustrates how detached the for-profit drug development establishment is from the business of protecting public health. After all, precious few patients in India are likely to enjoy the drug's benefits, however slim. At more than $3,000 for a course, the price of Xigris remains prohibitive, despite Lilly's successful lobbying of the government to drop custom duties on the drug.

If Xigris truly were the "only" drug to treat sepsis, as Eli Lilly India chairman Rajiv Gulati frequently tells the press, perhaps such mismatches between public health relevance and drug research might be tolerable. But it isn't. An alternative treatment that is both cheaper and safer exists: low-dose steroids. It languishes in unconfirmed obscurity. How many lives would have been saved had Lilly been compelled to devote some of its ADDRESS trial budget to establish the utility of steroids?

When faced with such questions, Kapadia bristled. "Every trial is always criticized," he said with frustration. His voice rose a notch and his speech quickened. "There is no trial that is perfect! There is almost no trial that can get every aspect of it right. I wouldn't say this trial would have more than its share of criticisms," he said. He paused, then added: "I really am unaware of any trial which has no criticism."[101]

8

Calibrating Ethical Codes

Peter Lurie's 1997 *New England Journal* paper and editor Marcia Angell's editorial decrying researchers' double standards for poor subjects—and likening them to the notorious Tuskegee Syphilis Study—opened years of tortured debate within the biomedical research community. "There have been gazillions of conferences and reports from national commissions and councils," said Johns Hopkins bioethicist Ruth Faden in 2001. "In the developing world, there's been a tremendous ratcheting up of interest in this question . . . of how to take account of politics and economic questions in research ethics." While the poles of the debate quickly emerged, with Lurie and Angell on one side and PhRMA spokespeople and FDA regulators on the other, most of the mainstream of the research community remained undecided. "We are struggling," said Faden. "We are reaching more consensus on conditions under which it is OK" to dole out substandard care in clinical trials, she said, but "increasing lack of consensus on whether it is alright in other circumstances."[1]

While the medical and bioethics press continued to appraise the intricate ethical complexities of the issue, a small battalion of researchers, led by FDA regulators and their advisers, attempted to seize the fluidity of the moment to shape ethical guidelines to their advantage. First, in the spring of 1999, Yale University physician Robert Levine, a key adviser in research ethics policymaking circles, circulated some proposed revisions to the Declaration of Helsinki, in advance of an upcoming meeting of the World Medical Association (WMA). How about, instead of insisting that subjects be assured of the "best proven" methods, Levine suggested, the declaration simply require that they be assured of the best proven methods "that would otherwise be available to him or her"?[2] The change would have altered the meaning of the edict entirely. With the addition of nine words, researchers could effectively wash their hands of any obligations to their subjects if they were poor or otherwise deprived.

Levine's proposal faltered at the October 2000 meeting. In light of the still simmering controversies over the mother-to-child HIV prevention trials, the WMA was moved to strengthen protections of research subjects rather than dilute them. They revised the declaration to reiterate that experimental treatments should indeed be tested against the best current treatment and underlined the dictum by pointing out that placebos were only permissible when there was no known effective treatment.[3] WMA secretary general Delon Human exulted in the new language. "We say almost explicitly . . . that if there is treatment, then you cannot give a sugar pill to the control group," he said to a *Washington Post* reporter after the meeting.[4] Ethics committees around the world referred to the Declaration of Helsinki when deciding on the ethical permissibility of trials; with the new language, they'd have vital ammunition to shut down placebo-controlled trials.

U.S. officials were irate. But it wasn't the public-health research community that was up in arms this time.

In 1975, the FDA had incorporated the Declaration of Helsinki into its rules for clinical trials conducted outside the United States, refreshing the regulations whenever the declaration was periodically revised.[5] Given the precedent, the agency would be expected to adopt this latest version as well. But the drug industry's ability to develop me-too drugs with little if any benefit over existing drugs—by testing them against placebos and conducting trials overseas—could come crashing to a halt if they did. Suddenly, ethics committees might start nixing trials of new allergy drugs when tested against placebos, or copycat drugs in other noncritical therapeutic areas.

"There are a lot of trials where the person isn't giving anything up and wants to be in the trial," the FDA's Robert Temple said to the *Washington Post*, offering hay fever and migraine drug trials as examples. "The declaration bars them, too. I think that's paternalistic." Not just that, either. Temple decreed the revised declaration "scientifically and ethically incorrect."[6]

In fact, just as Temple was doling out snippy quotes about allergy drugs to reporters, the agency was attempting to facilitate a placebo-controlled study in Latin America for a drug to treat fatally lung-impaired infants. There were already four such drugs on the market and the new drug, while easier to manufacture than its rivals, would likely provide no added benefit for patients, by the drugmaker's own admission. A trial that pitted the new drug against placebo seemed the only way to prove the drug worked at all and get it on the market, but no American parent would enroll in such a trial, risking their dying infant's life when already approved alternative drugs were available to them. The solution the company proposed was to run the trial at a poor hospital in Latin America instead. In January 2001, the FDA's Division of Pulmonary and Allergy Drug Products held a workshop to weigh the pros and cons of the proposed trial: "Use of placebo-controls in life threatening diseases: is the developing world the answer?" they dubbed the session.[7]

Peter Lurie, who had by then taken up a full-time position at the health watchdog group Public Citizen, raised a stink and forced the FDA to can the idea. Temple was miffed. "There is a certain satisfaction that everybody feels that this trial isn't happening," he said. But "those people [who would have been in the study] don't seem to have gained by this maintenance of principle." After all, the company was willing to upgrade decrepit hospital facilities in the developing country site to state-of-the-art. "Half of the people would have gotten surfactant and better care" than they would have otherwise, noted Temple. "The other half would get the better care."[8]

In the spring of 2001 the FDA announced that in defiance of two decades of precedent it would not be adopting the latest version of the Declaration of Helsinki into its regulations.[9]

Emboldened by the FDA's circumvention of the undesirably strict Declaration of Helsinki, U.S. researchers and bioethicists attempted a similar dismantling of the even stricter rules governing NIH research on human subjects.

Unlike trials aimed at FDA approval, which can get away with host country ethics reviews alone, NIH rules require that scientists procure ethics approval for their studies both in the United States and the host country. In November 2000, the National Bioethics Advisory Commission (NBAC), set up in 1995 to advise the U.S. government on ethical issues in biomedicine, started to make noises about dropping the requirement. In a draft version of a 2001 report on clinical trials in developing countries, the NBAC recommended that for overseas research, ethics reviews abroad would suffice on their own.[10]

NBAC planned to recommend this change despite evidence in the commission's own report that such overseas reviews would be unlikely to stop trials no matter how they measured up to the declaration's edicts. NBAC researchers had found that in Morocco, for instance, there were no ethical review committees, and "the Ministry of Health does not feel that it is necessary." Turkish officials had "serious reservations" about setting up ethics review committees. Researchers in Haiti said there had been no ethics committees in their country until 1999. Researchers in Uganda revealed that "the notion of an unbiased, uninvested review committee" was still "quite new" to the country. In an NBAC-commissioned anonymous survey, researchers active abroad had been startlingly frank about the ethics committees in developing countries that oversaw their trials. "Whatever happens to the patients, they don't care too much," one said. Ethics reviewers are "more concerned about the money," researchers told NBAC; "they have no control at all";

"they are looking [at] technical [issues] . . . and money, how much are you getting"; and "it is a political approval . . . more about whether we would be spies or . . . real researchers." The people in charge of the committees "have no idea about this. They just know [ethics] is a word."[11] Overall, one-quarter of clinical trials conducted in developing countries went through no ethical review whatsoever, the survey found.[12]

And yet, in its final April 2001 report, the NBAC's recommendations were, for the most part, noncommittal. On most of the thornier ethical issues confronting researchers, NBAC recommended simply passing the buck to local ethics committees. Researchers should try to provide "established effective treatment" whether or not it is routinely available, the NBAC opined, but if they don't, they should explain themselves to their ethics committees. Researchers should make "reasonable, good faith efforts" to provide study drugs to subjects after trials end, but if not, again, they should simply present their justifications to their ethics committees. On the question of whether researchers should capture both domestic and foreign ethics approvals, the NBAC recommended that researchers do get both—unless U.S. officials decided that the foreign site was sufficient on its own.[13] The NBAC report, noted Yale's Robert Levine approvingly, "put the world on notice that they [U.S. researchers] don't intend to comply" with the revised Declaration of Helsinki.[14]

In the summer of 2001, an industry-funded outfit, the Drug Information Association, held its annual meeting in Denver, Colorado. The FDA's Temple joined Caroline Loew, a spokesperson from the industry lobby group PhRMA, in attacking the WMA's Delon Human in front of a standing-room-only crowd. According to an account of the meeting circulated by a prominent bioethicist, Temple was scathing. The declaration "doesn't look like a group of suggestions that are worth discussing," he said. "It looks like a set of principles to be observed. And it says that every doctor has to observe these or he's not a good person."

Loew went straight to the heart of the matter. According to Loew, GlaxoSmithKline, Pfizer, and Merck had all had clinical trials banned by ethics reviewers because of the new Helsinki requirements. "Sooner or later it will be practically impossible to perform placebo-controlled studies for therapeutic confirmatory purposes," GlaxoSmithKline and AstraZeneca scientists wrote in a trade journal in 2001. "Indeed, it is already now increasingly difficult." If forced by ethics committees to test their new drugs against already available therapies, "improvement of therapy by degrees"—that is, copycat drugs—"will become impossible," they said.[15] "What we're seeing is important, ethical clinical research being disrupted," Loew said, "with the end result that access to innovative new medicine is deferred."[16]

Loew also aired the industry's objections to Article 30 of the declaration, which requires that research subjects should be assured access to whatever beneficial intervention is identified in the study, and Article 27, which requires that all results from clinical trials be published publicly. Human was overwhelmed. He announced he would convene a work group to reconsider the placebo restriction. His plan was to have "direct meetings with those who are critical," he said.[17]

In the fall of 2001, under pressure from the FDA and PhRMA, Human and the WMA issued a hasty retreat. The WMA revised the declaration yet again, the once elegantly concise document now appended with a wordy footnote "clarifying" the placebo rule. According to the footnote, "in general" placebos should not be used when proven therapy exists, but if placebos are necessary "for compelling and scientifically sound methodological reasons," or when the condition for which therapy would be withheld is minor, then they were "ethically acceptable."[18]

Lurie was outraged. "Where . . . is the footnote explaining in greater detail how informed consent should be obtained? Or how ethics committees should be constituted? Or how conflict of inter-est should be reduced or eliminated?" he railed in a 2003 letter to *Human*.[19]

The Helsinki dilutions didn't stop there, either.

Industry scientists stepped up their complaints that the Decla-ration of Helsinki's requirement that study subjects be "assured" of the best intervention as identified in the study was too onerous. "Firstly, none of the methods used in the study may be found to be suitable," Merck's Laurence Hirsch and Harry Guess wrote in the *British Medical Journal*.

> Secondly, a single study can rarely identify "best" treat-ment. . . . Thirdly, a new drug or device may not be approved until several years after the end of a trial. Consequently, pro-viding as yet unapproved treatment to trial participants on completion of the study may conflict with local regulations. Fi-nally, an offer to provide treatment that is otherwise unavail-able on completion of the trial might be considered an undue inducement to potential participants.[20]

"It is unrealistic and misleading to suggest that [drugmakers] can ensure access to drugs for any given population," seconded a paper by PhRMA. "Only local governments, not pharmaceuti-cal companies, can make decisions about initial, and particularly ongoing, access to new drugs. . . . There is a need first to estab-lish an appropriate infrastructure (e.g. roads, transportation, electricity, and water supplies)." Requiring such magnanimous gestures would surely bar drug companies from taking on re-search into new drugs for those diseases that public health advo-cates continually complained were neglected, the PhRMA paper warned.[21]

On cue, the WMA again convened a working group—this time to draft new language weakening the declaration's requirement that patients be assured of study drugs after trials end. In Septem-ber 2004, Helsinki gained another wordy footnote, clarifying that posttrial access to study drugs didn't have to be "assured," but merely "identified" and "described" before trials begin.[22]

With influential institutions such as UNAIDS, the National Bioethics Advisory Commission, and the WMA on record supporting double standards in medical research, other groups chimed in as well, including the Council for International Organization of Medical Sciences and the European Group on Ethics in Science and New Technologies. According to the new ethics regime, if there is solid scientific reason to believe trial subjects will not be harmed and can possibly benefit, then researchers should feel free to lower their ethical standards for impoverished patients. True, the new consensus might "create an insidious double standard that accepts for the poor what it rejects as unethical for the rich," defenders noted in a 2004 *Journal of Medical Ethics* paper, but "even if the position is not the optimal ethical standard, it is at least not clearly unethical."[23]

Ironically, one of the poster children of the standard-of-care debate—Jay Brooks Jackson's trial pitting nevirapine against placebo and ultra-short course AZT in preventing HIV infections in infants, a study condemned as unethical by Lurie—had meanwhile fallen out of favor. In September 2003, Jackson published his final report on the 012 trial, reporting on how the infants who survived the trial had fared eighteen months down the road. Although the nevirapine had saved more babies from HIV infection compared to the ultra-short course of AZT, it made no difference in saving their lives. After eighteen months the same proportion of babies had died in both groups. It wasn't clear why, but the fact that their HIV-burdened mothers—who did not receive antiretroviral therapy after the trial ended—had died might have had something to do with it.[24] Jackson said he would be checking up on the children again. He expected more of the toddlers in the AZT group to die in a few years' time. "HIV takes *time* to kill babies," he pointed out matter-of-factly.[25]

But why bother with single doses of nevirapine anymore, anyway? New York University's HIV researcher Karen Beckerman asked in the accompanying editorial. American patients had rightly shunned nevirapine as monotherapy back in the early 1990s because of its tendency to produce resistant strains of the virus. In 2001, Jackson's colleagues noted that nearly 20 percent of the women who received even a single dose of the drug had developed resistant strains of HIV. Likewise, if the infants exposed to the drug contracted HIV because the drug failed to work for them, or because their mothers passed on the virus through breast milk, they'd likely harbor resistant strains of the virus and find themselves dangerously limited in the kinds of therapies they might be able to take.[26] The entire class of nevirapine-like drugs could be rendered useless as AIDS treatments for them, Beckerman pointed out.

Combination antiretroviral therapy would both greatly decrease the chances of their babies catching the bug and would save the lives of mothers. It would also save the babies even if they did get infected—just as it had in the United States for years. With prices finally within reach, and lingering doubts about the ability of impoverished people to faithfully adhere to the regimen vanquished, there was no longer any need for "suboptimum" preventive techniques, she wrote. Single-dose nevirapine and other such second-rate solutions "no longer have a justifiable place in the front lines of global struggle against HIV/AIDS."[27]

Just as Helsinki was diluted in order to allow the kinds of trials that had brought the world single-dose nevirapine to prevent HIV infection in infants, the scientific consensus in favor of that treatment started to turn. In July 2004, South African health officials advised clinicians to stop administering nevirapine as an HIV prevention drug.[28]

Today AIDS researchers continue to justify giving substandard care to their test subjects in developing countries, in places where local standard of care is comparably poor. The trials Jackson planned in 2003 to launch in China were illustrative. Most revolved around experiments upon intravenous drug users, some of the most downtrodden people in Chinese society, their contaminated needles the source of at least half of the HIV infections in the country. The best current methods of helping intravenous drug users—clean needles and substitution drugs such as buprenorphine and methodone, for example—are routinely administered in Western countries. Not so in China, at the time Jackson planned to launch his studies. There, before 2004, the government had been known to throw illegal drug users into hospitals, force them into hard labor, and even execute them.[29]

And so, in Jackson's studies, the best proven methods would not be on offer. In one study Jackson would enroll Chinese intravenous drug users, comparing how some given nevirapine to prevent HIV infections fared against others given nothing but placebo.[30] In another he'd simply enroll them in a trial and count how many came down with HIV. In yet another he'd offer them all counseling, but give buprenorphine to only some and track how many became infected with HIV compared to those given placebo. None of the subjects who contracted HIV during the course of the trials would get antiretroviral therapy from the researchers. The Chinese government didn't offer it either.[31]

In 2001, NIH officials had suggested that Jackson might consider offering all of his Chinese subjects antiretrovirals and substitution therapies, treatment that would undoubtedly save many of their lives. Jackson objected. "American-style treatment programs are impractical at this point in China," he said. "It's unrealistic—even unethical—to think that we could provide Western standards of care to everyone in the world."[32]

In 2004, he was proved wrong, when the Chinese government announced it would offer free HIV testing to everyone in the country and antiretroviral treatment to all who needed it.[33] In 2005, officials announced their intention to legalize the use of methadone to treat intravenous drug users and step up needle-exchange programs. Meanwhile, the World Health Organization added both methadone and buprenorphine to its list of "essential medicines," drugs so crucial to public health that they should be available to all.[34]

Whether or not Jackson would be able to conduct his trial with nevirapine in China—as of 2005, the trial was in limbo—the arguments so staunchly forwarded in its favor had crumbled fast indeed.

VaxGen's trials of its tepid HIV vaccine in the United States and Thailand had, by early 2003, predictably failed. A smaller trial of an Aventis vaccine had a similarly weak showing, interim results revealed in 2002, leading researchers to give up on their plans for a larger trial testing the vaccine in the United States. And yet, in September 2003, NIH researchers chose to plow ahead with a trial that had been planned before the bad results: a massive trial in Thailand of a combination of the two failed vaccines.[35]

Critics such as Cornell University's John Moore and AIDS advocacy groups Treatment Action Group and Gay Men's Health Crisis complained loudly. Such data would likely render papers, grants, and scientific satisfaction, but had only a tenuous link to the search for an effective vaccine, they said. Many earlier vaccines had proven effective without scientists ever figuring out how they worked at all. But the researchers exhibited a steely determination to extract some usable data from the trial.[36]

By early 2005, ten thousand of a needed sixteen thousand subjects had been rounded up for the vaccine trial. Would the thousands of Thai subjects be informed that between the conception of the trial and its start date, both halves of the experimental vaccine they were being given had been shown ineffective? Local newspapers seemed oblivious, predicting that "the AIDS vaccine work programme will definitely be a success."[37] Lancet editor Richard Horton asked one of the safety monitors of the trial about "the propriety of continuing" the experiment. The monitor's response was evasive, as Horton later described in the New York Review of Books. "Good question," the monitor said, smiling anxiously.[38]

At the same time, Thai AIDS activists watched prevention campaigns in the country shrivel. "We spent millions of dollars for this no-hope project rather than spending that money on providing antiretroviral drugs for patients," complained one.[39]

As double standards in research ethics for poor people become increasingly acceptable in the research community, new arguments rationalizing the stripping down of subject protections have come into vogue. A popular one dismisses concern about defenseless test subjects as paternalistic. Nobody is forcing Thai sex workers or Chinese drug users to enroll in these experiments, goes the argument. They've decided for themselves. "You can't treat them as incapable of pursuing their own ends," says Temple. "They are not cavemen; they are just not rich."[40] In other words, informed and voluntary consent, that cornerstone of research ethics, offers sufficient protection, even for the most powerless. To the sick, poor subjects lining up at their clinic doors in Asia and Africa, clinical researchers might now echo used-car salespeople and the like: caveat emptor.

9

The Emperor Has No Clothes: The Vagaries of Informed Consent

Neisseria meningitidis is generally a placid sort of bacterium. Sluggish and round, it tends to quietly reside in the back of peoples' throats, minding its own business.

But every ten years or so, across a stretch of Africa from Ethiopia to Senegal, something different happens. Perhaps people have lost their immunity. Perhaps the bug has evolved into a more sinister form. Whatever the cause, during these episodes, when the dry air comes and *Neisseria* escapes in tiny, coughed-out droplets, the guest turns wild. *Neisseria* speed through the bloodstream of its new hosts—mostly children—finally reaching the meninges, those crucial membranes covering the brain and spinal cord, where it triggers a deadly inflammation.

Vomiting, high fever, and mental confusion follow. Around 80 percent of those sickened with *Neisseria*'s meningitis die, some within hours. During epidemics, tens of thousands might perish in a matter of months.[1]

One of the largest recorded outbreaks of epidemic meningitis occurred in 1996. The first reports trickled out of Nigeria in January. The next month, the numbers shot up. By March, the eruption was in full force, and emergency response teams from the Nigerian ministry of health along with the World Health Organization, UNICEF, and Médecins Sans Frontières rushed to Nigeria to dispense eight million doses of vaccine for those still well and powerful antibiotics to the ill. Another ten million vaccines were on the way.[2] Among those Nigerian children lucky enough to receive a rapid IV infusion of antibiotics, the chance of death would plummet to around one in ten.[3]

It didn't take long for news of the outbreak to reach Pfizer headquarters in chilly southeastern Connecticut, where it fell upon pricked ears. The company was racking up proof that its experimental broad-spectrum antibiotic Trovan worked on everything from gonorrhea to bronchitis and pneumonia, a potential $1 billion blockbuster in the making.[4] It seemed a golden opportunity to prove Trovan's mettle had fallen into the company's lap. In the United States, only about three thousand people contracted meningococcal meningitis every year.[5] In Nigeria, Pfizer could test Trovan on hundreds of untreated patients in a few weeks. If the FDA could be convinced that the drug worked for meningitis in these Nigerian kids, they could effectively break open the entire pediatric market. Pfizer's Scott Hopkins, MD, quickly drafted a protocol for a quickie experiment.

The news of the brewing plan alarmed Pfizer's infectious disease specialist, Juan Walterspiel. Walterspiel knew of his employer's eagerness to deliver the new bug fighter in convenient oral form rather than the usual injections proffered by competitors; to see how an oral formulation worked, the trial would administer Trovan in a tablet or a spoonful of syrup to some of the Nigerian children. But sending a drug into the body via the mouth is a circuitous route compared to shooting it straight into a vein, and Walterspiel knew that a rampaging *Neisseria meningitidis* can kill people fast. That's partly why the WHO recommends the use of injected antibiotics to counter meningitis outbreaks.[6] Plus, these kids in Nigeria weren't just facing one pathogenic microbe: they were malnourished and reeling from concurrent epidemics of measles and cholera. What if the bug overwhelmed them before the pills and syrup could be absorbed?[7] Their blood would be on the company's hands.[8]

But, according to allegations contained in a later lawsuit, neither Hopkins nor the rest of his six-person team took Walterspiel's concerns seriously.[9] In April 1996, filled with faith in Trovan's prowess, Hopkins and his team boarded a chartered DC-9 headed for the outbreak's epicenter: the dusty northern Nigerian city of Kano. "We had to move quickly," Betsy Raymond, a Pfizer spokesperson, explained to the *Washington Post* reporter who reported on the trial in 2000.[10]

The facilities in Kano did not impress Hopkins. At the Kano Infectious Disease Hospital, aid doctors conducted mass vaccinations and treated the sick with shots of chloramphenicol, the cheap, off-patent *Neisseria*-killer recommended by the WHO.[11] Chloramphenicol had been developed in the 1940s and had fallen out of favor in the United States in the early 1980s, when it was found to cause fatal aplastic anemia in one out of thirty thousand patients.[12] "I wouldn't give my dog [chloramphenicol]," Hopkins said to the *Post* in 2000.

The Pfizer scientist set to work taking over a ward of the crumbling cinder-block facility for his Trovan test. A nurse at a triage desk would direct the stream of ailing patients stumbling into the hospital either to the aid workers or to the Pfizer test clinic, where Hopkins would offer what he considered to be superior treatment options. Around one hundred lucky children would get Pfizer's Trovan and another one hundred Roche's Rocephin, a brand-name meningitis drug approved in 1993.[13]

Like many drug companies taking their trials overseas, Pfizer hadn't fussed with filing an application with the FDA before jetting over to Kano. Pfizer's researchers knew that in terms of patient protections, all the company needed to do was follow the mostly philosophical edicts of the Declaration of Helsinki and the FDA would likely happily accept the forthcoming data. This wasn't a high-profile experiment funded with public money, but a proprietary experiment that few outside the FDA and Pfizer would probably ever review in detail. The only concrete requirements entailed acquiring approval from a local ethics committee and, of course, written evidence of the subjects' informed consent.

* * *

Underneath the layers of oversight fashioned to protect human subjects from harm in medical experiments lies a hard inner core, forged when the horrors of coerced human experimentation were finally laid bare after World War II. It is the subject's own informed and voluntary consent—the oldest and most universally accepted ethical standard in research. "Ultimately," wrote NBAC researchers in a typical formulation of the standard's centrality, "research can go forward only if participants understand what the research entails."[14]

Few researchers, however, ever bother to verify whether their subjects do, in fact, understand. It wouldn't be difficult. Medical researchers routinely double-check, duplicate, and re-analyze nearly every other aspect of clinical trials by means of a profusion of journal articles, conferences, workshops, and lectures. "Relentless scrutiny of details" could be said to be the research industry's motto. But in the area of informed consent, an atypical atmosphere of "don't ask, don't tell" prevails.

One survey found that while over half of researchers admitted that it would be a good idea to verify their subjects' understanding of experiments, a scant 16 percent had ever done so in their own trials.[15] Partly that's because when researchers have attempted to confirm the integrity of informed consent, the bedrock has revealed itself to be made of very soft shale indeed.

In standard practice, to "consent" a subject, the investigator holds a single meeting with a prospective participant, explains the trial and the consent form, answers a few questions, and passes over the form for a signature. It is a brief, legalistic exchange that satisfies sponsors, oversight committees, and regulatory authorities, protecting all concerned from liability. But the evidence suggests it does little to enlighten test subjects about the risks of experimentation. This comprehension gap is even wider in the case of Western-sponsored trials conducted in developing countries.

Indrek Kelder, an accountant from Estonia, wasn't even sure what drug he'd been given in the 1998 industry trial he participated in.

"Maybe it was written between all this mumbo jumbo," he offered to the *Washington Post*. His fellow trial subject, Estonia's Irme Petrimae, was similarly confused. "They told me something about skin disease," he allowed. "All these forms, and we didn't get any copies. I didn't like it . . . but it was too late to change our minds."[16] Despite having signed informed consent forms, no fewer than thirty of thirty-three Thai volunteers enrolled in one trial of an experimental HIV vaccine later said they shared the mistaken belief that "the vaccine they received was effective," according to a 1997 study published in the *Journal of the Medical Association of Thailand*.[17] In Haiti in 2002, when researchers turned around and quizzed subjects on the basic outlines of the HIV transmission experiment they had just agreed to, 80 percent flunked.[18] In a 1998 study in Brazil all subjects in a trial of an experimental contraceptive enrolled under the erroneous impression that the experimental intervention "would be good for them."[19]

Disturbing signs that test subjects' participation in trials is not particularly voluntary have also emerged. In a 1998 analysis by South African epidemiologists, more than eight out of ten South African women inducted into an HIV prevention trial, all of whom had already been through an informed consent process, professed to feeling coerced into remaining in the trial.[20] "Two little bottles of blood was taken from us without asking our permission," complained an HIV-positive South African woman who enrolled in a trial after being approached by a recruiter on her street.[21] A similar proportion of Bangladeshi women in a 1998 trial on iron supplements revealed that they had no idea they were free to abandon the experiment.[22]

The best evidence of voluntary, informed consent is when some subjects drop out or refuse to participate in a trial, researchers say. "That's a good sign," one noted to NBAC researchers. "They are able to refuse, they are free to refuse [to enroll]."[23] And yet, in NBAC's 2001 survey of researchers active in developing countries, 45 percent reported that their low-literacy subjects *never* refused to participate.[24]

"I want the money," explained Thai taxi driver Wivat Chotchat-
mala, a drug user who enrolled in one of VaxGen's HIV vaccine
trials.[25] "We continued to visit the distribution center" to participate in a U.S.-government sponsored trial of a new antimalarial
drug, said Kenyan villager Lucas Oyombe Otieno, "so as to enjoy
the free meals." Otieno and his fellow subjects had already
stopped taking the study drug because of its unpleasant side effects. "We would collect our drugs, pretend to swallow them, but
we would throw them away later," he told the *East African Standard* in 2004. "When they offered to provide us food, many of us
accepted to be used in the study," added Andrew Okal Seda, who
enrolled in a similar antimalarial drug study in Kenya. "Around
that time, there was widespread famine in the area."[26]

And the truth is that, contrary to the blithe pronouncements of
the NBAC and others that research can only proceed when subjects are informed and participate consensually, for some CROs,
uninformed, coerced subjects don't impede medical research at
all. On the contrary, unknowing, docile subjects make trials easier
and faster.

"Russian subjects don't miss appointments, they take all the required pills, they fill in the questionnaires and the diaries, and
only very rarely do they withdraw their consent. . . . Russian subjects do what their doctors tell them to do. What a phenomenon!"
a promotional article in the trade journal *Applied Clinical Trials*
gushed.[27] CROs routinely tout the "compliance" of their experimental subjects on offer, especially those in poor countries where
many patients are lucky if they can get a doctor to pay attention to
them at all. James Loudon, an executive from a CRO active in
China, encouraged drug companies to experiment on patients
there, not because the patients are empowered and informed, but
because "the Chinese are not that fully emancipated as in the U.S.
They are more willing to be guinea pigs," he said to CenterWatch
in 2002. "It's not like Japan, where it's difficult to get patients to do
trials, or they refuse at the last minute."[28]

It isn't technically difficult to ensure that even the most

unknowing, premodern, and illiterate subjects are informed and consensual partners in high-tech medical research. Scientific notions ingrained in Western society may be foreign to others, but they are not beyond comprehension. "You can do it, if you put in enough resources," says Anne-Valerie Kaninda, an aid doctor who treated meningitis-stricken children in the same Kano hospital where Pfizer conducted its Trovan test. "People are not as stupid as they are portrayed. I understand that it might be difficult to talk about informed consent when you are coming in with Western concepts of medicine, and there you have a mother with a sick child who doesn't know what a microbe is. But still, if you put in enough resources, with a translator you can still explain, 'You have a choice, either you go the regular way, or you come with us; we are testing.' . . . It means that whoever is conducting the trial has to put resources into that, with a lot of well trained people."[29]

Several simple methods have been shown to bridge the gulf between Western investigators and patients from developing countries. Researchers can take advantage of the fact that some patients in developing countries are more capable and inquisitive than their Western counterparts by virtue of having survived in more difficult, resource-constrained environments.[30] After subjects sign the forms, researchers can quiz them. Those with low scores can be counseled further, or dropped from the trial. Study staff can hold periodic meetings with subjects to answer questions as they come up and ensure their participation remains voluntary.[31] Researchers can hire local people to explain the study, by using pictures and diagrams, and references to local practices in agriculture or community life. They can launch educational programs about the experiments in the larger community. They can approach community leaders to help establish legitimacy first.[32]

If after all this, informed consent is still not achieved, then the prudent response might be similar to that taken when a piece of crucial equipment fails. The study, rendered untenable, is abandoned. Such practices might stymie some trials, but "not all knowledge is accessible," says bioethicist Jonathan Moreno. "It is one of the trade-offs between realizing there is a moral difference between people and lab rats."[33]

But in many cases, that is not what happens.

Instead, researchers and regulators profess defeat—and press on anyway. They try and they try, but getting impoverished, illiterate villagers to understand and consent to their experiments is simply very difficult, if not impossible, some insist. M. Upvall and S. Hashwani of Aga Khan University in Pakistan compared informed consent procedures in Pakistan and Swaziland for a 2001 *International Nursing Review* paper. According to their study, researchers were often forced to penetrate layer after layer of tribal hierarchy and corrupted bureaucracy in order to obtain informed consent. Sometimes they had to ask the village elders or the husbands of women participants first, or employ police escorts, or have tea and snacks, "regardless of the time it took." Plus, they had to struggle with the fact that some subjects don't have telephones, or permanent addresses, and may even be afraid to sign their names. Such findings on the barriers to informed consent "demonstrate the inadequacy and complexity of applying western-based concepts of informed consent to developing countries," Upvall and Hashwani wrote.[34]

It is a pointless exercise, some researchers insisted to NBAC analysts in an anonymous 2001 survey. In some African languages "there is no word for 'research' or 'science,'" one says. "There is no concept of an experiment or placebos."[35] "Informed consent is a joke," said another. "It is not possible to claim a person who has never heard of a bacteria or virus is informed about what a vaccine or drug is doing or how their participation fits into any such study."[36] Perhaps informed consent is just too Western a notion, they say. After all, "this concept of the consent of the individual, rights, and individual decision-making doesn't exist" in many authoritarian developing countries, one said. "People do what they are told, and people are told what to do."[37] In India, according to a 1996 *Journal of the Royal Society of Medicine* paper, physicians consider informed consent "an unnecessary ritual."[38] In Latin America, one doctor told the *Washington Post* in 2000, physicians were "against" informed consent. "Patients want doctors who say, 'Do this because I say so.' "[39]

Some industry researchers are even more forthright. They must mislead subjects because "if all potential adverse effects are listed in the informed consent, the patient will be scared away," as John C.M. Lee, a Bristol-Myers Squibb researcher working in China wrote. "One needs some flexibility in implementing" requirements for informed consent. Due to educational and cultural background, a complete written informed consent is very difficult to achieve. It is a very long-term goal that China follow the international standard in this area.[40]

Even regulators profess impotence. "We have requirements for informed consent," says the FDA's Robert Temple, but "I'm not going to tell you it is always well done. . . . Should there be more real-time interviews? Some ethicists talk about this. It is an area that needs attention. But we don't do anything about it immediately. We rarely go to a study that is ongoing."[41]

Not a single subject signed a form indicating his or her consensual participation in Pfizer's Trovan experiment in Nigeria. The children were too young to sign, the company said in its defense, and the parents didn't speak English, the language the form was in. But in addition, no witnesses attested to any verbal consent, if it was given at all.[42] According to Elaine Kusel, a lawyer who would later represent the Nigerian families involved, it wasn't. The subjects "had no idea they were part of any clinical trial."[43]

Despite Pfizer's apparent inability to acquire written evidence of consent, the researchers didn't throw their hands in the air and jet back home. They moved forward with their experiment anyway.

Researchers are often convinced they are helping their subjects, whether the patients know it or not. In the end, Pfizer lost the same proportion of children in their Trovan group as their Rocephin group, around 6 percent.[44] So, even with subjects later saying they were tricked into participating, the attitude of other Western researchers is cavalier. "I don't see the harm in it," said

UCLA meningitis expert Larry Baraff of the study. "It sounds like they all did well."[45]

But not everyone evaluates outcomes in the same way, which is, of course, the underlying logic of respecting others' right to choose in the first place. "It is kind of a colonial or imperial attitude, if you like," says prominent South African bioethicist Solomon Benatar. "There seems to be this idea that if you want to do a trial in Africa, and you want to set the same standards for that trial as you did in Europe or America, all you need to do is have the best proven drug. But the standard of care in a research study goes beyond the drug. . . . Until such time as you are paying the same amount of attention to the standard of informed consent, then I wonder why are you making so much noise about the drug? Is our mind-set framed by the pharmaceutical industry? Is our mind-set not framed enough by the conditions under which people live—and what it means to be treated with respect by a foreigner?"[46]

The FDA reviewed Pfizer's data from Nigeria in early 1997. They didn't question the statement indicating ethics committee approval. The fact that it had been backdated and the hospital in question didn't have an ethics committee at the time of the trial didn't emerge until 2001, after the *Washington Post* exposed the trial.[47] Nor did the agency have anything to say about the utter lack of evidence of participants' informed consent.[48] On the contrary, when regulators indicated to Pfizer that the Nigerian trial wouldn't fly, it wasn't because of these ethical violations: rather, there were "discrepancies" in the data. Despite it all, the agency went on to approve Trovan for fourteen adult uses, the largest number ever for a drug's initial approval.[49]

The complicity of regulators, industry researchers, and academic scientists in circumventing the requirement for informed consent is not limited to experiments conducted on unwitting, uncomprehending foreigners. Even in the United States, regulators have

long turned a blind eye to coercion and misunderstanding between subjects and researchers.

The first clause of the Nuremberg Code, that experimental subjects be "able to exercise free power of choice," indicated to most
countries around the world the impermissibility of experimentation
upon those forcibly restrained behind bars. And yet, when the 1962
amendments to the U.S. Food and Drug Act required that drug
companies suddenly experiment on scores of living bodies, the U.S.
prison population served as "almost the exclusive subjects" for
early drug trials, according to a 1994 federal advisory committee
report on government-sponsored human experimentation. Some
pharmaceutical companies even built their testing laboratories next
door to prisons to ease their access to the incarcerated masses.[50]

The practice of experimenting on prisoners only ended in the
1970s, when the Tuskegee study exploded onto headlines. In its
wake, public mistrust in all human experimentation ran so deep
that an influential 1974 *Scientific American* paper went so far as to
argue that all placebo-controlled trials were profoundly deceptive,
since some patients would think they were getting active treatments when in fact they weren't. "To permit a widespread practice of deception . . . is to set the stage for abuse and growing
mistrust," the paper argued.[51] Drug companies, sensing the change
in the wind, quietly disassembled their prisoner drug-testing facilities. "We were getting too much hassle and heat from the press.
It just didn't seem worth it," remembers an administrator from
one of Eli Lilly's test clinics at an Indiana prison.[52]

Despite the 1979 Belmont Report's clear statement that human
subjects must not be tempted into risky experiments by cash or
other benefits,[53] drug companies quickly found that offering a
modest sum to broke students and homeless people provided a
plentiful supply of recruits. Soon the industry's test clinics had
quietly migrated to the nation's university campuses. Today
Pfizer's new test clinic conveniently nestles next to Yale University; Bristol-Meyers Squibb's next to Princeton University; Glaxo's
next to Imperial College in London.[54]

Students and homeless people flock to the industry's gleaming facilities. For Ben Leff, a University of Chicago law student, becoming a guinea pig netted him "more money than I had ever made doing anything," he said. At a pay rate of around $100 to $200 a day, including room and board, "it's money for doing almost nothing," he exclaimed.[55]

Nineteen-year-old Traci Johnson took up experimentation to earn the $3,600 she needed to pay for a semester's worth of tuition and fees at Indiana Bible College in Indianapolis. The bible college recommended students apply for jobs at the local post office or Starbucks, for example,[56] but there was a better option just seven miles away from her school: volunteering as a research subject for experimental drug trials run by Eli Lilly. At $150 a day the job paid twice as much as the starting wage at Starbucks, and included board and a "hotel-like" room, not to mention a pool table, cafeteria, and rooftop sundeck.[57] Other volunteers said the experience was less like a job and more like a "mini-vacation." "It's like staying in a really nice hotel," one said. "The lobby view is gorgeous," added another.[58] Johnson could earn enough for another semester of school in less than a month.

In January 2004, Johnson checked into the Lilly clinic and enrolled in a study of duloxetine, an antidepressant in the same class—selective serotonin reuptake inhibitors (SSRI)—as Prozac. Over the following weeks clinicians gave her increasingly larger doses of the drug, up to six times greater than the recommended therapeutic dose, and tracked how she metabolized it.[59] When not involved in study activities, Johnson and the other drugged subjects watched television and shot pool.

Meanwhile, across the Atlantic, British medical authorities were banning the use of SSRI drugs in people under the age of eighteen. Six months before Johnson's enrollment in the trial, the FDA, sufficiently aroused, had ordered one of its researchers to investigate the growing body of evidence linking the drugs to suicidal behavior.

As Johnson started the trial, the researcher had revealed his findings to his superiors in the agency: people under eighteen years of age who took the drugs were twice as likely to engage in suicide-related behavior compared to those who didn't take them. The danger was greatest within four days of stopping the drug, he reported. The FDA decided to keep its findings secret.[60]

On or around February 3, the nineteen-year-old Johnson was taken off the duloxetine; the protocol called for placebos during the final four days of the study. Some subjects reportedly felt "uncomfortable" after being withdrawn from the drug, a Lilly doc noted, but not Johnson, apparently.[61] On February 6, she called her best friend on the phone, laughing and sounding happy, as her friend remembers it.[62] Johnson had, by then, earned $3,600 in the Lilly trial, enough to go back to bible school in the fall.

The next day she tied a scarf around the shower rod in her bathroom and hung herself.[63]

Two months after the FDA cleared the drug of any role in Johnson's death and approved it for marketing, it ordered makers of antidepressants, including Lilly's Cymbalta, to warn doctors that the drugs could increase the risk of suicidal thoughts and behavior in children and adolescents. By July 2005, the FDA had found a link between duloxetine and heightened rates of suicide attempts in adults as well: women taking the drug for relief from urinary incontinence.[64]

Some people have found they can eke out a meager living selling their bodies to industry science, flitting from center to center, enrolling in trial after trial for years at a time. Most such "professional volunteers" are students seeking to supplement their income, homeless people, or casually employed workers. "One guy in his forties had twenty-two kids and his girlfriend was pregnant," Leff recalls about a fellow trial participant. "He did it for the diaper money."[65]

For the research establishment, questions as to whether $200 a day is too much to offer to students and homeless people in exchange for their bodies, or whether such payments exploit the financial desperation of the poorest members of society, remain hazy and undecided. As the volume of Phase 1 trials expands virtually unhindered, such "ethical questions," intoned the National Institutes of Health's Neal Dickert and Christine Grady in a 1999 *New England Journal of Medicine* paper, "remain unresolved."[66]

Neither the country's ethics committees nor the FDA have much to say on the matter: "oversight of the recruitment of subjects is minimal," according to a withering 2000 Department of Health and Human Services report on the topic, "and largely unresponsive to emerging concerns."[67] Rather than acknowledge that they are buying access to human bodies for their trials, researchers tend to speak euphemistically. The "reimbursements" are small, they say: "We don't pay patients to do clinical trials," scoffed a clinical investigator at a Boehringer-Ingelheim research facility. "They get a fee for taking time out of their day and they get a fee for transport."[68]

And yet it is clear from such publications as *Guinea Pig Zero*, which calls itself "the journal for human research subjects," what brings eager volunteers to test clinic doors. "The pay rate is high-end and the studies tend to be long and lucrative," a *Guinea Pig Zero* review of one research center noted. "They pay you for the travel and there are no unnecessary visits or procedures." Little is mentioned about the mission of medical research, although the free laundromat, TV, and outdoor courtyard for dining all merit special attention.[69] But even the most outspoken subjects don't bother shattering the mythology that eases the investigator-subject relationship. As a researcher extracted her bone marrow, one subject recalls in a *Guinea Pig Zero* essay, "I just smiled and said I was glad to do my part for humanity."[70]

For Phase 2 and Phase 3 trials, healthy subjects are not sufficient and recruitment becomes a bigger challenge. For these trials, sick

people—patients—with the particular condition under consideration must be convinced to try out a new drug. With rich rewards
in extended patent exclusivity on offer for companies that test
their new drugs on children, sick kids and their parents must be
enticed as well.

As the competition for access to these sick bodies has increased, subtly deceptive practices have become the norm. The
problem lies in the fact that sick people are especially dependent
upon the advice and authority of their clinicians. They are ill, and
they need help. Generally, that isn't a problem, as doctors are
likewise enjoined by the Hippocratic oath to align their interests
with those of their patients. But that isn't the case in clinical trials. Here the doctor-investigator's first commitment is no longer
to the patient: it is to the data, whether the experiment helps the
patient or not.

Of course, it is possible to fully inform patients about the differences between therapy and experimentation, and to acquire
their voluntary consent. In earlier decades, when drug companies
recruited sick patients for experiments by contracting with university hospitals, such distinctions were less problematic. Patients
visiting research and teaching facilities had already implicitly
signed on for cutting-edge, sometimes experimental methods.

But things started to change when the industry quit academia
in favor of quick trials run by for-profit clinical trials companies
such as CROs. CROs don't fuss with pointy-headed university
types. They approach doctors out in the community. The trouble
is, when a patient visits her local doctor at the clinic on Main
Street, she is expecting proven therapy, not experimental research,
and the difference isn't trivial, for doctors or patients. And as the
pressures on community physicians to enroll ever greater volumes of patients at ever greater speeds grows, the incentive to
blur the lines between therapy and experimentation intensifies.[71]

As HMOs pressure doctors to cut corners and spend less
money and time on their patients, CROs offer doctors as much as
$12,000 for simply enrolling a single patient into a trial,[72] and they

provide high-tech equipment. The work, after all, involves helping companies produce new drugs that help people. Today private practices, medical centers, and clinics actively compete for
CRO contracts, scrambling for "a larger piece of the pie," as University of California professor of medicine Thomas Bodenheimer
wrote in a 2000 *New England Journal of Medicine* paper.[73]

In a reversal of earlier marketing efforts that advertised a
clinic's medical services for patients, clinics now advertise their
patients for industry experimentation. "Looking for trials!" ran
one typical ad cited in the 2000 Department of Health and Human
Services report. "We are a large family practice with 5 physicians
and 3 physician's assistants . . . and a computerized patient data
base of 40,000 patients. . . . We can actively recruit patients for any
study that can be conducted in the Family Practice setting."[74]

Some CROs even offer generous bonuses for those who can lure
patients into trials fastest or in the greatest volume, dangling perks
such as an author byline on a prestigious journal article. According
to a clinician quoted in the Department of Health and Human Services report, if a bonus was available for a physician after enrolling,
say, thirty subjects and the doc had twenty-nine already, "you could
bet that the site would get the 30th subject."[75] Even the eminent former surgeon general, C. Everett Koop, got in on the action, negotiating a deal with Quintiles to funnel patients visiting his popular
health-related Web site to the company's clinical trial sites.[76]

By 2003, CROs were raking in nearly $70 billion a year finding
human bodies for experiments,[77] some of them growing even
larger than their drug company clients.[78] New companies have
emerged as subcontractors to the exploding CRO industry. "Our
specialty is delivering qualified, motivated patients to health care
professionals who use your product, and to your clinical trial
sites," the patient recruitment firm ThreeWire advertises.[79] "Your
subjects are out there somewhere," Clinical Solutions, another recruitment firm, writes on its Web site. "We can find them."[80]

Do doctors thus enticed into providing test subjects bypass the
strictures of informed consent? It's not unheard of. In 1997, two

physicians from a medical college in Georgia were indicted for faking the medical records of their schizophrenic patients in order to enroll them in lucrative drug trials.[81] In the late 1990s, a University of Oklahoma–sponsored physician misled melanoma patients enrolled in a vaccine trial that it was the "best vaccine out there," and failed to inform them of adverse effects, sparking a congressional inquiry.[82]

In 1996, a surgeon at the University of South Florida tricked sixty subjects into a study of an experimental cutting tool.[83] In 1999, eighteen-year-old Jesse Gelsinger died in a Phase 1 study of a gene-transfer technique at the University of Pennsylvania; neither Gelsinger nor his parents had been informed of previously documented adverse events or the salient fact that the investigators who presided over Gelsinger's care in the experiment had financial interests in the company that was commercializing the technique. In 2001, a healthy volunteer, Ellen Roche, died from the inhalation of a chemical irritant; she hadn't been informed that the compound had already been proven dangerous to humans in previous studies. (In this case, the investigator hadn't known either.)[84]

According to government investigators, most patients are by and large unaware that their blood draws, urine samples, and hospital visits are being pored over quite so intently by people other than their own doctor. When the letters and phone calls roll in, asking them if they'd be interested in participating in a clinical trial for their diabetes or arthritis, it probably seems like fortuitous serendipity. Later the patient is approached by his familiar physician, holding court in his familiar white coat in his familiar examining room. But this time the doc is conducting an experiment rather than providing care.

Surveys showed that the overwhelming majority of patients— nearly 90 percent, according to some studies—consent to experimental trials under the mistaken impression that they will personally benefit from them. Despite dutifully signing their informed consent forms, two-thirds have no idea what the purpose of the trial they joined is, researchers have found.[85] "The idea that altruism is an important consideration for most patients with cancer," wrote one lymphoma sufferer, a former industry researcher, "is a figment of the ethicist's and statistician's imagination."[86] Instead, the *American Journal of Bioethics* affirmed in 2003 that the therapeutic misconception—patients' mistaken belief that experimental techniques will help them—"is not the exception, but the rule in modern research."[87] "I guess everybody looks at it as grandeur, you know," explained a subject of a placebo-controlled trial to Harvard Medical School researchers. "Saying, 'wow, I'll take this pill and everything will stop.' " "I was positive it [the trial] would help me," another trial subject said. "I was positive going in and I was positive through the whole thing."[88]

Recruitment firms and drug companies—even medical facilities—encourage the confusion. They describe the human participants they need not as subjects of an experiment but simply as patients. One cancer center wrote on its Web site that "a clinical trial is just one of many treatment options" available—as if a clinical trial were, indeed, the same as medical therapy.[89] Physician investigators don't generally inform their subjects of the generous recruitment fees and stock options they acquire after patients sign on the dotted line.[90] Nor are subjects generally told that the biggest trials requiring the most patients typically stand the least chance of helping them. (The larger the trial, the lower the manufacturer's expectation in the beneficial effect of the new drug.[91])

"My oncologist is really encouraging me to sign up for the Herceptin trial," a breast cancer patient wrote on a support group Web site in 2003, referring to new trials of the blockbuster breast cancer drug. "He's actually trying to 'scare' me into it by going on and on about my 'great risk.' I am terrified now that if I don't do it, I am basically choosing to die from this."[92] The physician's subtle coercion ("enroll or you'll die") and misinformation ("I know this drug will help you") worked: the woman ended up enrolling in the trial, desperately hoping that she didn't get randomized into the placebo group.

*   *   *

In their defense, physician investigators point out that manipulating patients' beliefs has always been integral to the art of medicine. Doctors can relieve pain in patients, for example, by simply telling them they are receiving an effective painkiller, even while giving them placebos.[93] Studies show that when doctors offer a meaningful diagnosis and benign attention, and reassure the patient that healing could occur, they do heal many of their patients, whether or not the therapy they prescribe is effective or not, as determined by randomized controlled trials.[94]

Because of this, the requirements of informed consent virtually guarantee that doctors' potency as healers is diminished. The more rigorously patients understand the risks of experimental methods, the less likely they are to benefit from their faith in the doctor or the drug. As Mumbai clinical researcher Farhad Kapadia noted, "You know, you have an international standard [for the] consent form, and it is pretty explicit. When I use a drug in someone who is not in a trial, I don't go to all these lengths to explain. I say, 'there are good and bad effects, and generally I think it will help, and if you can afford it we'll go for it.' But here, I've got to explain everything. I don't know if they [the patients] feel put off, but they are not so comfortable. If you tell someone there are twenty side effects, they'd be more worried about taking aspirin, rather than if I say, 'Take this, it is good for your heart.' "[95]

Not only is informed consent thus an impossible standard, uninformed consent is practically a necessity, some say. "Patients hear what they want to hear and they don't hear what they don't want to hear," commented one surgeon casually at a gathering of CRO executives in 2003. So getting informed consent from a patient is "an exercise in futility."[96] Around the room, heads nodded. Nobody reads the informed consent forms, claimed UCLA meningitis researcher Larry Baraff in an interview. "They look at you, they think you are a decent person, you explain it the best you can, and they just sign the thing."[97]

It wouldn't be difficult for the FDA to require that investigators not only provide written evidence of consent, but actually prove that such consent is truly informed and voluntary. But instead, the agency routinely accepts what amounts to drug companies' word that their patients have been adequately informed. According to agency whistleblowers, its medical officers are actively discouraged from looking too closely at the consent forms.[98]

Nobody, it seems, wants to stand in the way of new trials and slow the pace of medical progress by pointing out that informed consent is an emperor with no clothes. "Why do we keep using informed consent despite knowing it doesn't really work?" asks bioethicist Jonathan Moreno. "We haven't got an alternative."[99]

That may change. In 2001, thirty Nigerian families filed *Abdullah v. Pfizer*, a class action suit claiming that Pfizer violated the Nuremberg Code in its 1996 Trovan experiment in Nigeria. According to the lawsuit, the company failed to inform the children or their parents that Trovan was experimental and "that they were free to refuse it." But whether the justice system will be able to correct for regulators' and researchers' laxity on informed consent is as yet unclear. The suit, initially dismissed by the U.S. District Court in Manhattan, was remanded back to the court on appeal in October 2003. As of 2005, the case had yet to be heard.[100]

10

Tipping the Scales

Most of us rarely have a say in how clinical trials are run, or where. And yet we, as members of society, are the ones who collectively bestow upon researchers their conditional privilege to conduct experiments on humans. Without our tacit blessing, the whole business lacks legitimacy.

And so, just as ethics committees evaluate the risks and benefits of individual trials, society must evaluate the risks and benefits of the entire business of human experimentation.

The trouble is, there's a tendency in the United States to minimize the risks of research while lionizing its benefits, which complicates a fair appraisal of the balance between the two. In popular coverage of research, investigators tend to describe the risks of their work in microscopic detail, constrained by time and place—the test subjects might suffer some skin rash, or some fatigue, or anemia, researchers might allow. Rarely are broader risks—such as the possible undermining of human rights or the hijacking of scarce health care resources—mentioned. That's fair enough, except that on the topic of benefits, investigators tend to be expansive and speculative, including the experiment's hypothetical effect on thousands and even millions of other people, not just in the near term, but over years and even decades.[1]

In a typical formulation, the National Bioethics Advisory Commission wrote that "research has resulted in improvements to health, created valuable new products for everyday living, provided the capacity to sustain cleaner environments in a rapidly industrializing world, and facilitated better personal and family relationships." An impressive litany, to be sure, and doubtlessly true. But what about all the research that has resulted in less sparkling developments, such as, say, the atom bomb, DDT, and the silicon breast implant?

Faith in the benefits of scientific research remains untarnished despite its failures. The "war on cancer," launched by President Nixon in 1971, provides an example. While deaths from heart disease and cerebrovascular diseases had already peaked in the United States, cancer's death toll continued to grow during the 1970s.[2] Evidence that curtailing smoking could stanch the unfolding epidemic had emerged by 1956.[3] Yet instead of devoting billions to stamping out smoking, or fingering other environmental triggers for cancer, the U.S. government spent $5 billion between 1971 and 1978 to search for new drugs to administer to ailing cancer patients. A flood of new drugs was duly unleashed, but five-year survival rates for cancers of all kinds increased from 39 percent in the 1950s to just 41 percent by the late 1970s. (The war on cancer, FDA commissioner Donald Kennedy said to *U.S. News and World Report* in 1978, had become the nation's medical Vietnam.[4])

Faith in the benefits of biomedical research is even stronger when it involves problems faced in the developing world. "It takes half a second to see how much more burdened the developing world is with ill health and disability," says Johns Hopkins bioethicist Ruth Faden. The great need in developing countries, for Faden and others, is not primarily more infrastructure or education but more research. "What we need if anything is more health research in the developing world, not less," Faden says.[5]

In January 2003, the Bill and Melinda Gates Foundation, now the world's leading private funder of international health research, launched an ambitious initiative to tackle the most destructive health problems plaguing the developing world. To wit, Gates funds research into new vaccines that don't need to be refrigerated, or require multiple visits to scarce health clinics; development of a single plant species that provides multiple micronutrients; and new chemicals that control disease-carrying insects, among other things.

Research into cheap, easy solutions like these, if implemented, would help countless people in poor countries. But vaccines that don't need refrigeration, shots that only need to be given once, and single plant species that might provide adequate nutrients do little to extract the poor from their health care–deprived environments bereft of clean water and electricity. On the contrary, in effect they engineer ways for people to survive in them indefinitely.[6]

If money, time, and resources were unlimited, a bit of blind optimism wouldn't matter much. But in a world of scarcity, exaggerating the benefits of research can be downright dangerous. "There are many millions of people around the world who don't have access to the scientific advances of the last hundred years," notes South African bioethicist Solomon Benatar. "In fact, if you go to any developing country and ask the people there, they'd say, 'Well, we're not so much interested in doing research. We're interested in having access to the things that you have already found that work! Why come here to ask research questions when actually what we need is what has already been discovered! Why should we believe that this new research is going to benefit us if the old research doesn't benefit us?' "[7]

The scale that Western research advocates often use to weigh risks and benefits of trials is often skewed by a general fuzziness over who takes on the risks and who gets the benefits, too. Such was the case in a series of confrontations during 2004 and 2005 between Cambodian and Thai patient-advocates and Western AIDS researchers and their allies.

In recent years, with HIV vaccine research in the doldrums, AIDS prevention researchers have explored a new approach: the use of antiretroviral pills to ward off infection. Nevirapine and AZT prevent newborns exposed to HIV from getting infected, the thinking goes; what if other antiretroviral drugs, given once a day, could do the same for adults exposed to the bug? People engaged in high-risk activities could pop a pill every day and save themselves from infection, just as Western travelers down antimalarial drugs to ward off malaria before venturing into tropical swamps.

The idea of preventing HIV infections in this way has already been put into practice in a limited fashion. In 1996, the CDC recommended that health care workers exposed to HIV on the job, through inadvertent needle sticks or the like, be given rapid treatment with antiretroviral drugs, even before it was known if they were infected.[8]

Launched in 2001, Gilead Science's Viread (tenofovir) seemed a good candidate for this use. Unlike other antiretroviral drugs, tenofovir is effective even when taken just once a day, doesn't have to be taken with food, and has few toxic side effects.[9] By 2004, the CDC, NIH, and the Gates Foundation were planning major new trials testing the new theory. A small Phase 2 trial involving a few hundred subjects would take place in San Francisco and Atlanta. There, researchers would organize subjects into three separate groups; two would get tenofovir or placebo right away, while the other one would simply get counseling, so that researchers could carefully track whether the treated subjects emboldened by hope in the drug grew more lax toward other protective measures, always a risk in trials of new HIV prevention methods. Since these studies weren't designed to measure how well tenofovir protected subjects from the contagion, it wouldn't be necessary for researchers to rack up sufficient HIV infections in the placebo group in order to have sensible results.[10]

Not so in Asian and African countries, where researchers planned to launch straight into large-scale Phase 3 trials without waiting for the Phase 2 results. While the U.S. study was ongoing, the CDC would enroll 1,200 men and women in Botswana and 1,600 intravenous drug users in Thailand.[11] The NIH would test the drug on 960 Cambodian sex workers in Phnom Penh.[12] The Gates Foundation would sponsor trials of 1,200 high-risk women in Ghana, Cameroon, and Nigeria.[13]

As in all research into new HIV prevention methods, the subjects would be vulnerable to slacking off on proven effective safeguards such as condoms and clean needles. Around half of all the high-risk subjects in the trials wouldn't receive the hypothetical protection of tenofovir either, as they'd get placebos. Once again, in the case of the Thai drug users, the CDC wouldn't provide clean needles. The Thai government condemned such provision. Its reviled 2003 campaign against illegal drug use had resulted in widespread human rights violations, including two thousand extrajudicial murders, according to Human Rights Watch.[14]

In the summer of 2004, ACT UP Paris and a Cambodian sex workers' advocacy group decried the trials at an international AIDS conference, spilling fake blood on Gilead's displays and surrounding the speakers' podium angrily.[15] According to the activists—and hotly denied by researchers—the subjects were being enrolled by blackmail, the counseling offered to them was minimal, and investigators refused to take responsibility for treating any of the subjects who became ill under their watch.[16] Such unfortunates would "have to rely on Cambodia's low standard of healthcare and limited access to antiviral drugs," as the *Wall Street Journal* reported.[17]

Alarmed, the Cambodian prime minister shut down the trial.[18] Four months later, Thai AIDS activists starting making noises about the tenofovir trials in Thailand as well. Drug users in Thailand suffered an HIV infection rate of 50 percent and were violently oppressed by the government. How could researchers possibly protect their best interests, as required by the Declaration of Helsinki? They couldn't even provide clean needles, the single best known measure of HIV prevention for intravenous drug users, a "particularly egregious departure" from Helsinki standards requiring researchers to provide all experimental subjects with the "best current" methods.[19] A month later, ACT UP Paris surrounded the Cameroon embassy in France, condemning the Cameroon tenofovir trial as unethical too.[20] By February 2005, the Cameroon Ministry of Health had suspended the study.[21] In

March 2005, researchers themselves canceled the tenofovir trial in Nigeria.[22]

The AIDS research community was roiling. "It's a disgraceful day for AIDS activism," said Mark Harrington, an AIDS activist with the New York–based Treatment Action Group.[23] "These forces threaten to derail future trials," complained two AIDS-vaccine NGOs, Global Campaign for Microbicides and the AIDS Vaccine Advocacy Coalition, in a statement. "The cost is paid in people's lives—the lives of those who might benefit from new technologies or treatments."[24] Sure the experiments entailed some risk, but look at the benefits, they said. Tenofovir prophylaxis is "perhaps the single greatest near-term hope for the prevention of AIDS," the *Wall Street Journal* reported.[25] If tenofovir worked, it could "revolutionise AIDS prevention," echoed the *Financial Times*.[26]

But for whom?

Researchers hadn't determined whether sex workers in Cameroon really would pop a prescription pill every day for the rest of their working lives, or if so, whether they would be able to afford it. "Would it be a sustainable preventive tool? We don't know enough about that," allowed Mitchell Warren of the AIDS Vaccine Advocacy Coalition.[27] Maybe it would be. Western researchers had thought Africans wouldn't take ARVs or use condoms, but they did. On the other hand, it wasn't peevish to suggest that maybe it wouldn't. Gilead announced that it would sell the drug at cost in poor countries—85¢ compared to $12 per pill in the United States[28]—but according to Médecins Sans Frontières spokespeople, the company had neglected to apply for marketing approval in poor countries, making the nice-sounding offer "a virtual one."[29] What's more, the most obvious precedent—antimalarial pills to prevent malaria—had done little to prevent millions of people in developing countries from that scourge. Those drugs are enjoyed almost exclusively by Western travelers, not by people who live in malarial regions.

It isn't that quantifying the potential benefits lies beyond the ken of science. In fact, researchers had already delved into the

questions of how the drug, if proven effective, could be administered and to whom; what clinicians might do if the drug were not
fully effective; how subjects might afford to buy sufficient quantities of the drug; whether they were likely to take them faithfully
or not; and what would happen to them if they didn't. The only
problem was, that analysis had been conducted for California.[30]

Meanwhile, the risks of the trial appeared to build. In February
2005, CDC scientists revealed that all the monkeys they had dosed
with tenofovir had gotten infected with simian HIV anyway.[31]
The AIDS Vaccine Advocacy Coalition continued to tout the benefits of the trial to developing countries as an article of faith. "It
could be used by millions of people," the group wrote in defense
of the besieged trials. "The world loves biomedical answers."[32]

Could activists in developing countries be blamed for wonder-
ing: which part of the world?

Fully realizing the promise of medical research, whether inflated
or not, requires a gargantuan effort for which researchers can't, on
their own, bear responsibility. They just provide the data. Patients,
clinicians, health care companies, and national governments,
among other entities, are the ones who have to translate scientific
results into action. But there are other benefits of clinical trials—
more limited in scope but more tangible—that investigators can
easily facilitate, such as making sure that trial subjects have access
to the study drug (if proven effective) after trials end.

And yet, anecdotal evidence suggests that both industry
and academic researchers are generally reluctant to take on the
responsibility. That's the government's job, not theirs, they say.
"It is hard to ask the sponsor of the trial to make up for the fact
that the country isn't providing treatment," says the FDA's Robert
Temple. CROs wash their hands of the entire affair. "It has to do
with the commitments the companies can make, which varies
from trial to trial," says Wurzlemann, adding, tepidly, that "it is a
matter of concern among everyone."[33]

Academic researchers are among the most reluctant to fulfill such obligations. Jay Brooks Jackson is one of the best-funded researchers at Johns Hopkins University. "We ship tons of stuff every week" to clinical sites overseas, he says. "Test kits, reagents, software, I mean it is just endless, it is endless." But Jackson does not provide antiretroviral drugs to the patients in his prevention studies who become infected with HIV while he is studying them. "We refer them for symptomatic care and that sort of thing; it is sort of like what you would do in 1985 [in the United States]. . . . Over time, when you've worked in these countries, you just realize that this is sort of the way it is," he says.[34]

Academic researchers worry that if they insist on providing study drugs to the subjects of their trials, their funders will lose interest in footing the bill for the trial. They also contend that promising patients drugs after trials end might be too good of a deal: patients would throw caution to the winds and join the trial regardless of the risks. Better, in that case, not to make any promises. "Only governments can provide long-term care guarantees," AIDS vaccine researcher and advocate Seth Berkley argued.[35]

Anyway, FDA officials, CRO execs, and industry researchers who run trials abroad argue, just looking at the potential benefits of the drug in a trial is too simplistic a way to evaluate all the benefits that might accrue to the participants and their society from taking on a clinical trial. Even when experimental subjects don't benefit from the study drug, they likely benefit from the extra medical attention they'd be bound to receive in a trial aimed at getting a drug approved by the FDA. "You see, patients are very cared for in trials," said Nadeem Rais, a diabetes specialist who conducts industry trials in Mumbai, India. And these medical services are not only free; in many trials, subjects are even paid to participate.[36]

A 1999 study, for instance, found that patients enrolled in randomized controlled clinical trials survive better and with fewer complications than those getting care outside research protocols.[37] "Companies need to do clinical trials in developing countries, because the trials bring benefits to the patients," says HIV researcher Arthur Ammann, who has tried to convince companies to do more trials in developing countries. "They get special attention. . . . And they provide potential therapy for those patients."[38]

"Patients who go into these trials are getting really, really good care," said Macé Schuurmans, a lung specialist who has conducted industry trials in Switzerland and at South Africa's Stellenbosch University. He says his South African patients are very grateful to him for conducting these trials on them. "In an affluent country, you give the patient the best treatment you know of, and it is usually available. Here, [in South Africa], you have to decide if you can do five chemotherapies, and you've got twenty patients. Which five will get that chemotherapy? . . . If you see the queues in hospitals . . . they'll wait the whole day. People go there, they cough, and maybe cross-infect themselves. They have to wait to see the doctor, they have to queue to get the medicines. [But if they get into an industry trial], if they wait for the doctor at all, they get tea, they get to look at television and it is quite nice. . . . The patient is really very happy. They say, 'Gosh, I'm really happy this happened to me.' "[39]

There are intangible benefits that accrue to the facility running the trial, too, which may eventually help local patients in other ways, Schuurmans and others say. Sometimes poorly equipped clinics will get a new machine or two for use during the trial and to keep afterward. Clinicians might get specialized training that they can later use to treat patients. During its Trovan test, Pfizer upgraded facilities at Kano Infectious Disease Hospital with high-tech equipment.[40] The company even doubled one lab technician's salary for helping with the trial, the *Washington Post* reported.[41]

"It generates quite a lot of hard-earned money," says Schuurmans, money that can be used to treat patients or conduct public health–oriented research.[42] "We got some equipment, and they didn't ask for it back," after an industry-sponsored trial ended, says Mumbai-based cardiologist Yash Lokhandwala. "Per patient recruited for the trial, they give a sum that goes to the hospital; it is, like, 15,000 rupees per patient, so if you get one hundred patients, that comes to fifteen lakhs of rupees [around $33,000] for the hospital."[43]

Doctors and nurses might learn about cutting-edge new drugs and the latest techniques. After all, "distribution of wealth and knowledge is unequal," Wurzlemann, the CRO doc, said. "Sharing that knowledge helps make the world more fair." It is unlikely that American doctors and patients would tolerate such trade-offs, but elsewhere clinicians profess gratitude. The placebo-controlled trial of nitazoxanide, which resulted in thirteen deaths in Lusaka's University Teaching Hospital in 2000–2001 and failed to ensure a later supply of an approved drug, "was a good experience for Zambia," affirmed University Teaching Hospital clinician Mary Ngoma.[44]

For others, a few token machines and payments do not always compensate for the diversion of precious health care resources away from treating patients. Lokhandwala conducted clinical trials for multinational drug companies while working at an over-burdened public hospital in Mumbai. He recalls: "For these trials, everything has to be maintained, documented, kept in the cup-board for three years. The fridge has to be maintained at the same temperature. If the temperature goes a little bit more or less, you have to immediately alert them, and you have to stop the trials until the repairman comes, and so on. Suppose you break an am-pule, you have to keep that broken part, to make sure you keep it for the study monitors to show that you had two or three. Who is going to do all this? I had my usual duties and, in addition, this trial was a big headache for me. . . . Here in clinical work everyone is overworked, and then you tell someone to spend their time on paperwork!"[45]

Clearly, reading the scale on risks and benefits is no straightfor-ward task. It depends on whom you ask, when, and in what context. "The idea that one can pronounce on the ethics of some-thing today and that will be correct forever," says Benatar, "would seem to suggest that ethics is like a cookery book. If you want to make cookies, you can make them with a recipe and they will always look and taste the same. The ethics of international re-search are infinitely more complicated than that."[46]

The clinical research establishment manages the complexity by essentially leaving it to the experts. "There is sensitivity in some parts around who can speak on ethical issues," affirms South African human rights activist and physician Leslie London. The general idea is that the appropriate venue for discussing risks and benefits of clinical trials is not the front page but cloistered ethics-committee meeting rooms and the pages of academic journals, where bioethicists and researchers delve into the complexities of a single trial at a time. It's a piecemeal, microscopic approach that isn't particularly well-equipped to grapple with how trials, in the aggregate, may exploit subjects' poverty, undermine human rights, or misallocate resources. "You get sort of 'well you balance this and you balance that and this is important,'" says London.

"And you never get a straight answer."[47]

Conclusion

Listen long enough to biomedical researchers, as I recently did at a multidisciplinary scientific conference, and you will doubtless hear admiring commentary about human experiments of days past, when daring trials free of onerous regulation produced spectacular results. Such experimentation, the research scientist will say, is unfortunately no longer possible "due to ethical concerns."

Due to ethical concerns. I heard the phrase at least a few times over the course of a single week-long conference. It is an interesting construction, which seems to be almost exclusively reserved for biomedical transgressions. It's hard to imagine anyone talking about indentured labor, or oil spills, or corporate embezzlement as not being possible "due to ethical concerns." Those things are simply considered morally wrong and socially illegitimate, and are punishable by law. But when clinical researchers deceive patients, exploit their poverty, or divert scarce resources away from their care, it isn't considered an unalloyed bad. The main business of medical research—improving health, saving lives—overshadows it. The exploitation and human rights violations are just side effects.

Subduing these "side effects" requires mothballing the mythology around medical research that sets them up as "side effects" in the first place. As bioethicist Solomon Benatar explains, "Research being done in developing countries . . . is not really for the benefit of those people [the subjects]. It may happen to be, for the few people lucky enough to get into the trial. But the reason the researcher is coming to that country is more often than not because somebody is willing to pay for the study. Somebody wants an answer to a question. The data is valuable either academically or commercially."[1]

In other words, the main business of clinical research is not enhancing or saving lives but acquiring stuff: data. It is an industry, not a social service. The people who sponsor and direct clinical trials do it for the data, not to please patients or to help bolster ailing health facilities, although they may point to these side effects to justify their activities. Their motives don't make them corrupt or mercenary, either, just regular, self-protective humans like the rest of us.

But if clinical research is a self-serving industry, then there's no reason to allow it special leeway, to look the other way when it bends and even breaks the rules. If we think that trial subjects should be informed and their participation should be consensual, we should require that informed consent gets checked and confirmed. If it's impossible, then we should require the research be stopped. We should require that the deals for subjects— access to study drugs after the trial ends, for example—be fair and good right here and now, not in some speculative future when prices fall, or poverty ends, and other people apply better solutions.

Such requirements, which could be incorporated into FDA rules, would be logical correctives to the profit-driven, competitive industry that clinical research has now become. But that begs the question as to whether we really want to accommodate this model in the first place.

Rather than simply dispelling the myths, we could start to demand that drug companies and medical researchers actually live up to them. The promise of medical research is that it will alleviate ill health and save lives, but clinical researchers only take on a tiny slice of that job: getting the data. When it comes to implementation, shoulders are shrugged: that's someone else's job. The disconnect might be acceptable for basic science, but if we want medical research to truly alleviate ill health and save lives, then we have to hold it accountable when it renders little more than interesting papers and "me-too" drugs, whether it does so ethically or not.

Achieving this kind of accountability is no easy task. The public has no mechanism for setting priorities in research in the first place, no way to articulate what it is that we most want from medical research, and how we would use it if we had it. Aside from a few targeted programs, either the market decides and research goes into whatever drug companies think will sell, or sponsors decide on a case-by-case basis and whichever grant applications look most interesting get funded. Imagine instead a systematic review and a robust, independent, open public debate on where medical research has gotten us thus far and where it is that we want it to take us, not just among specialists and advocates, but all of us. It is hard to say where such an exercise might lead. Perhaps we'd see that research on the shelf has little meaning. Poor countries may well prioritize the implementation of old research over the pursuit of new experimentation.

Opportunities to exploit the gap between the haves and have-nots would shrivel.

There are obvious pitfalls in these suggestions. Drug companies can easily find loopholes in stricter informed consent and other rules. Researchers can easily mount convincing arguments that millions will die if research is delayed or burdened with greater accountability. But there is one suggestion for slowing the body hunt that is fairly airtight, and that is to require that new drugs prove themselves better than already available ones, not just better than nothing.

This would trigger a profound shift in drug development and the clinical research it entails. Not only would it maximize the potential for drug trials to render public health benefits, but such trials would prove less risky for subjects, too. Investigators would, by necessity, provide all of them with active treatments. More important, higher FDA standards for new drugs would cut much of the fat out of the drug industry, favoring companies that produced useful new drugs rather than hypermarketed copycats. The pace of new drug development would inevitably slow, as would the concomitant hunt for bodies. The competitive urgency that leads researchers to dilute ethical standards or transgress them entirely might start to abate.

Of course such a change would likely require an act of Congress and the drug industry would fight it tooth and nail, enlisting sympathetic patient groups to support them. We're not nearly there yet. But to get us on the road, we can start supporting drug developers that are already doing something similar: nonprofit outfits that develop drugs aimed at public health. If public and nonprofit drug companies can show they can develop worthwhile drugs efficiently, public confidence in the idea of making medicines not as a business but as a public health effort might grow. It may not seem so radical, then, to raise the bar on FDA rules, too.

It used to bother me that people could be so squeamish about human experimentation but yet have no problem capitalizing on the products it renders. It is the same kind of "not in my backyard" attitude that sends toxic waste and open-pit mining to Asia and Africa while Americans enjoy disposable plastics and aluminum foil. But I've come to believe it signifies something deeper: an understanding that there is something unsettling about using people for their tissues, blood, and metabolism. Turning the body into a thing rightly offends our sensibilities about what it means to be human. Experimentation depersonalizes us: trial subjects no longer have humor, style, habit, ideas. And we like to think of ourselves as more than just mushy machines.

But medicines are not just commodities, they are social goods, and their development requires experimentation on humans. So long as that remains true, we need to find ways to do it right, and to do it fairly.

Notes

Preface

1. Daniel Callahan, *What Price Better Health? Hazards of the Research Imperative* (Los Angeles: University of California Press, 2003), 3.

2. Jon Cohen, *Shots in the Dark: The Wayward Search for an AIDS Vaccine* (New York: W.W. Norton, 2001), 100.

3. Ibid., 251.

4. Julie Schmit, "Costs, Regulations Move More Drug Tests Outside USA," *USA Today*, May 16, 2005; Marc Kaufman, "Clinical Trials of Drugs Fewer, Study Says: Report Also Notes Decline in Number of Principal Investigators in U.S.," *Washington Post*, May 4, 2005, A2.

1: Clinical Trials Go Global

1. See "Drop in Death Rates for Diseases Treated with Pharmaceuticals, 1965–1996," available at www.quintiles.com, citing U.S. National Center for Health Statistics 1998.

2. John Wurzlemann, "Presentation on Eastern Europe," in Globalization of Clinical Trials panel, Maximizing Clinical Efficiency Phases conference (Washington, DC, October 9, 2003).

3. Mark McLellan, "The Current Status of Clinical Trials," in Maximizing Clinical Efficiency Phases conference (Washington, DC, October 9, 2003).

4. Andrew Pollack, "Three Universities Join Researcher to Develop Drugs," *New York Times*, July 31, 2003.

5. David Horrobin, "Are Large Clinical Trials in Rapidly Lethal Diseases Usually Ethical?" *The Lancet*, February 22, 2003, 695−97.

6. Stan Bernard, "The Drug Drought: Primary Causes, Promising Solutions," *Pharmaceutical Executive*, November 2002, 7.

7. Bonnie Brescia, "Better Budgeting for Patient Recruitment," *Pharmaceutical Executive*, May 2002, 86; Andrew Pollack, "In Drug Research, the Guinea Pigs of Choice Are, Well, Human," *New York Times*, August 4, 2004.

8. The bubble of goodwill burst within weeks, when a faulty batch of vaccine was released, infecting 220 children with polio. Laurie Garrett, *Betrayal of Trust: The Collapse of Global Public Health* (New York: Hyperion, 2000), 330. The public recoiled in horror. Salk's vaccine, it was later revealed, also contained monkey tissue, a potential source of other pathogenic viruses, some of which could have triggered certain cancers. Anita Guerrini, *Experimenting with Humans and Animals: From Galen to Animal Rights* (Baltimore: Johns Hopkins University Press, 2003), 129.

9. Garrett, *Betrayal of Trust*, 330; Sarah Marie Lambert and Howard Markel, "Making History: Thomas Francis, Jr., MD, and the 1954 Salk Poliomyelitis Vaccine Field Trial," *Archives of Pediatrics and Adolescent Medicine*, May 2000, 512; Marcia Meldrum, " 'A Calculated Risk': The Salk Polio Vaccine Field Trials of 1954," *BMJ*, October 31, 1998, 1233−36.

10. Kathleen B. Drennan, "Pharma Wants You: Clinical Trials Are Agencies' New Proving Ground," *Pharmaceutical Executive*, April 2003, 83−84.

11. Dan Moskowitz, "What Stops Cancer Patients Enrolling?" *Scrip*, November 2002, 13.

12. In the original randomized, double-blind, placebo-controlled trial some subjects with metastatic breast cancer would get ninety minutes of infusion with Herceptin. Other, equally ill women would get ninety minutes of infusion with some inert substance. Then the researchers would watch to see which group got sicker faster. Patients couldn't have been less interested in participating. A year later the trial was still underenrolled. To entice more patients into the trial the CRO running the Herceptin trial dropped the placebo group. Despite the fact that for all anyone knew Herceptin could have been worse than a placebo, enrollment skyrocketed 500 percent over the original lethargic rate. "Patients

were also much more willing to travel to the clinic each week to receive treatment," the CRO exulted on its Web site. See www.covance.com/clinical/content/pg_clin_case-onc.html. Interview with Dennis DeRosia, 2001.

13. Horrobin, "Are Large Clinical Trials in Rapidly Lethal Diseases Usually Ethical?"

14. Harsha Murthy, "The Use of Innovative Strategies in Patient Recruitment: Best Practices and Success Stories from Pharma and Biotech," Maximizing Clinical Efficiency Phases conference, (Washington, DC, October 10, 2003).

15. Horrobin, "Are Large Clinical Trials in Rapidly Lethal Diseases Usually Ethical?"

16. Bernard, "The Drug Drought."

17. Roy Porter, *The Greatest Benefit to Mankind: A Medical History of Humanity* (New York: W.W. Norton, 1997), 67.

18. Thomas Bodenheimer, "Uneasy Alliance—Clinical Investigators and the Pharmaceutical Industry," *New England Journal of Medicine*, May 18, 2000, 1539–44.

19. Ibid.

20. See Quintiles Web site at www.quintiles.com.

21. Sonia Shah, "The Globalization of Clinical Research," *The Nation*, July 1, 2002.

22. Public Citizen, "Comments on the Draft Health and Human Services Inspector General's Report," Washington, DC, July 5, 2001.

23. U.S. Department of Health and Human Services, *Report of the Office of Inspector General: The Globalization of Clinical Trials: A Growing Challenge in Protecting Human Subjects*, September 2001, iii.

24. "In an average year, we estimate that approximately 1,140 foreign clinical trials . . . are conducted under IND review and oversight. . . . [W]e can . . . estimate that 575 non-IND foreign trials are conducted annually for eventual submission to FDA for research or marketing applications." From "Human Subject Protection; Foreign Clinical Studies Not Conducted under an Investigational New Drug Application," *Federal Register*, June 10, 2004.

25. U.S. Department of Health and Human Services, *Report of the Office of Inspector General: The Globalization of Clinical Trials*, iii.

26. Marc Kaufman, "Clinical Trials of Drugs Fewer, Study Says," *Washington Post*, May 4, 2005, A2.

27. Julie Schmit, "Costs, Regulations Move More Drug Tests Outside USA," *USA Today*, May 16, 2005.

28. Pfizer press release, reprinted from "India Hub to Lead Pfizer's Clinical Studies in Asia," *Times of India*, October 3, 2003; "The Trial Trail," *Business India*, March 3, 2003.

29. See www.quintiles.com/Corporate_Info/Regions/south_africa_and_india.

30. Interview with Bradley Logan, October 2003.

31. "Treating Study Volunteers as Customers," *CenterWatch Industry Reports*, March 2003, 1, 4.

32. Yuri Raifeld and John Wurzlemann, Globalization of Clinical Trials panel, Maximizing Clinical Efficiency Phases conference (Washington, DC, October 9, 2003).

33. See www.quintiles.com/Corporate_Info/Regions/south_africa_and_india.

34. "Lifting India's Barriers to Clinical Trials," *CenterWatch*, August 2003.

35. Pfizer press release, October 3, 2003; "The Trial Trail."

36. Jeetha D'silva, "AstraZeneca, Glaxo to Make India R&D Hub," *Economic Times*, September 8, 2003.

37. "GSK Cuts Costs with More R&D Abroad, Electronic Data Capture," *Drug Industry Daily*, November 6, 2004.

38. Tufts Center for the Study of Drug Development, "CROs Provide Gateway to Worldwide Clinical Trial Recruitment Efforts," *Impact Report*, July/August 2003.

39. Ad for Neeman Medical International, from *R&D Directions*, July/August 2003.

40. "Success with Trials in Poland," *R&D Directions*, July/August 2003, 28; Zheng-ming Chen, "Organizing Large Randomized Trials in China: Opportunities and Challenges," *Drug Information Journal* 32 (1998): 1193S–1200S; Diego Glancszipigel, "Clinical Trials in Latin America," *Applied Clinical Trials*, May 2003, 38; Sergei Varshavsky, "Discover Russia for Conducting Clinical Research," *Applied Clinical Trials*, March 2002, 74; "A Billion Dollar Clinical Research Opportunity Lies in India," *BioSpectrum*, August 19, 2003.

41. Interview with Carel Ijsselmuiden, September 4, 2003.

42. Malcolm Potts, "Thinking about Vaginal Microbicide Testing," *American Journal of Public Health* 90, no. 2 (February 2000): 190.

43. Without quinine neither the British nor the French would have been able to colonize malarial Africa—while the natives could survive the disease, it stopped Europeans dead in their tracks more effectively than any resisting army. Porter, *The Greatest Benefit to Mankind*, 163–66, 230, 233, 465–66, 482.

44. Porter, *The Greatest Benefit to Mankind*, 237.

45. Meredith Fort, Mary Anne Mercer, and Oscar Gish, eds., *Sickness and Wealth: The Corporate Assault on Global Health* (Cambridge, MA: South End Press, 2004), 22.

46. London surgeon John Snow established that cholera spread via contaminated water in 1854; a British army surgeon proved that mosquitoes transmit malaria in 1897. Porter, *The Greatest Benefit to Mankind*, 412–13, 468–70.

47. Sheldon Watts, *Epidemics and History: Disease, Power, and Imperialism* (New Haven, CT: Yale University Press), 167–212.

48. A British army surgeon had discovered the wily parasite that causes malaria, lurking in the bellies of blood-thirsty mosquitoes back in 1897. Within a few decades, by draining the standing water pits where mosquitoes bred, screening windows so the bugs couldn't get into bedrooms, and similar methods, malaria had been all but eradicated from much of the United States and northern Europe. The U.S. military had likewise eradicated malaria from tropical Panama, on account of their desire to build a canal through that country's narrow jungle-covered isthmus.

But Western aid doctors, now led by the newly formed World Health Organization and tasked in 1948 with the business of "applying modern remedies" to all the countries of the world, did not seek to undertake such time-consuming and costly measures. By then, an "easy relief" from malaria had been discovered: the insecticide DDT. DDT was cheap and easy to apply, and had already saved the lives of millions of soldiers sent to the battlefield with a can of the stuff in hand. Practically indestructible, a spritz of DDT could kill adult mosquitoes as well as their offspring, and its powdery residues would continue the carnage even years later. In 1955, the WHO boldly declared that if given sufficient quantities of DDT, it would eradicate malaria from the face of the planet.

Between 1958 and 1963, the United States generously funded the WHO's anti-malaria campaign. The disease was successfully eradicated from southern Europe, and greatly lessened in India, Malaysia, and Sri Lanka. But as was clear from as early as the mid-1950s, malaria-carrying *Anopheles* mosquitoes could quickly become resistant to DDT, which was being vigorously applied not just by the WHO but by farmers everywhere, encouraged by Western officials overseeing the World Bank. In 1962, the toxic chemical's environmental effects, from cancers and fish kills, were damningly indicted in Rachel Carson's groundbreaking book *Silent Spring*. "Almost overnight," remembers one entomologist, DDT became " 'the elixir of death.' " A year later Congress refused to allocate funds to the WHO program. After the plug was pulled on DDT, the denizens of malaria-ridden regions faced a massive return of the mosquitoes, this time shorn of their low-level immunity to malaria. Porter, *The Greatest Benefit to Mankind*, 468–91; "Development and Constitution of the W.H.O.," *Chronicle of the World Health Organization: 1947*, vol. 1; Giancarlo Majori, "The Long Road to Malaria Eradication," *The Lancet*, December 18, 1999; Susan W. Fisher, "Once-Admired Chemical DDT Has Instructive History," *Columbus Dispatch*, June 11, 2000, 6B; Laurie Garrett, *The Coming Plague: Newly Emerging Diseases in a World Out of Balance* (New York: Penguin Books, 1994), 47–53.

49. Garrett, *The Coming Plague*, 42–46; Porter, *The Greatest Benefit to Mankind*, 472–91.

50. The bank's drastic pronouncements quickly drowned out the suggestions of World Health Organization officials and even local governments' health departments. In a single year, the bank could offer $2.5 billion for health care projects in indebted countries, making it—not the WHO nor local health officials—the developing world's most influential authority on health policy. The entire annual budget of the World Health Organization, in contrast, dawdled around $900 million throughout the 1990s. Fort, Mercer, and Gish, eds., *Sickness and Wealth*, 128, 205.

51. Jim Yong Kim et al., eds., *Dying for Growth: Global Inequality and the Health of the Poor* (Monroe, ME: Common Courage Press, 2000), 93, 113, 143, citing Mebelo K.N. Mutukwa et al., "The Structural Adjustment Program in Zambia: Reflections from the Private Sector," in Kapil Kapoor, ed., *Africa's Experience with Structural Adjustment*, World Bank Discussion Paper 288, 1995, 73–87.

52. Sarah Sexton, "Trading Health Care Away? GATS, Public Services and Privatization," Corner House Briefing 23, July 2001.

53. Kim et al., *Dying for Growth*, 158–65.

54. Similar "shock therapy" and "structural adjustment programs" transformed post-Soviet Russia, which in 1992 embarked on a risky plan to radically transform its state socialist system into a market-based capitalist economy. Formerly free public hospitals and clinics suddenly demanded exorbitant fees for their services to people newly out of work, bereft of housing and food subsidies previously supplied by the state, and faced with skyrocketing inflation. By 1995, about half of all Russians had fallen into poverty, while a tiny fraction of the population made a killing. Russians were dying faster than they were replenishing their numbers with healthy babies, "a demographic pattern usually seen only in times of war, famine, or plague," noted health economists Mark G. Field, David M. Kotz, and Gene Bukhman. Before the economic meltdown diphtheria had practically disappeared in Russia, with just 903 cases reported in 1989. By 1994, diphtheria had taken almost 40,000 Russians. The paternalistic, authoritarian Soviet TB control program—mandatory screening and months- and years-long exile for the infected in drafty sanatoriums—had effectively stifled tuberculosis, the caseload dropping by 5 percent to 7 percent every year. The program collapsed in the early 1990s, but little took its place save aging X-ray equipment and spotty drug supplies for the few who could pay for it. By 1998, no fewer than 2.5 million of Russia's 148 million had fallen prey to the ancient scourge. Worse, almost a third of all tuberculosis victims in Russia's prisons were beholden to a particularly nasty multidrug-resistant form. Kim et al., *Dying for Growth*, 158–65; Sarah Sexton, "Trading Health Care Away?"

55. By the end of the 1990s the AIDS pandemic and tuberculosis had effected a drastic turnabout in some African countries. A slow, steady march forward in life expectancy had been reversed. Kim et al., *Dying for Growth*, 5, 106–8.

56. Ibid., 208.

57. The company is now the largest employer on the continent of Africa. Sonia Shah, "Coke in Your Faucet?" *The Progressive*, August 2001, 29–30.

58. The business of penetrating new markets took on such import that Western officials willingly undermined public health protections in foreign countries if they appeared obstructive. In the mid-1990s, for example, U.S. State Department officials forced Guatemala to gut a widely praised law that had saved the lives of scores of infants. The law banned the use of images of chubby babies on infant-formula packaging, thus reducing the allure of a product that was too often reconstituted with dangerously contaminated water. When baby food manufacturer Gerber objected, state department officials threatened Guatemala with trade sanctions, and Guatemalan officials gutted the law, exempting Gerber and other baby-food importers from its strictures. "Prepared Statement of Lori Wallach, Global Trade Watch," House Ways and Means Committee, Trade Subcommittee, Federal News Service, August 5, 1999; Gary Gardner and Brian Halweil, *Underfed and Overfed: The Global Epidemic of Malnutrition*, Worldwatch Institute Paper, March 2000, 33.

59. In Western countries the transition from the hardscrabble malnourishment of the hunting-gathering days to today's drive-through, fast-food cornucopia had occurred over centuries, with the happy result that communities were able to control infectious diseases spread by poverty and hunger before facing the maladies of richly calorific diets, including diabetes, obesity, and heart disease. In developing countries no such time lag exists. In many countries, what nutrition experts call the "nutrition transition" is taking place within a single generation. Benjamin Caballero and Barry M. Popkin, eds., *The Nutrition Transition: Diet and Disease in the Developing World* (London: Academic Press, 2002), 140–41.

60. Joint WHO/FAO Expert Consultation, *Diet, Nutrition, and the Prevention of Chronic Diseases* (Geneva: World Health Organization, 2003).

61. Kim et al., *Dying for Growth*, 208.

62. Caballero and Popkin, eds., *The Nutrition Transition*, 165.

63. Ibid., 130, 160, 165, 183.

64. Sarah Boseley, "Clinton's AIDS Plan Snubs Bush Plan," *The Guardian*, April 7, 2004.

65. Robert Radtke, "India Must Steer a Middle Path on Generic Drugs," *Financial Times*, March 24, 2005, 13.

66. Audrey R. Chapman et al., eds., *Human Rights and Health: The Legacy of Apartheid* (Washington, DC: American Association for the Advancement of Science, 1998), 20.

67. Interview with Marta Darder, November 13, 2003.

68. Porter, *The Greatest Benefit to Mankind*, 621.

69. Interview with Robin Pelteret, November 9, 2003.

70. This figure includes drug-trial funding from the Medical Research Council of South Africa and the Gates Foundation along with drug company contracts. The rationale is that the drug industry funds will subsidize public health–oriented research. Interview with Robin Pelteret, November 9, 2003.

2: The Placebo Control

1. Phillip J. Hilts, *Protecting America's Health: The FDA, Business, and One Hundred Years of Regulation* (New York: Alfred A. Knopf, 2003), 225.

2. Ibid., 229.

3. Many Phase 3 failures are due to the fact that drug companies expect their drugs to be more effective than they are, and thus fail to enroll sufficient numbers of patients necessary to show their drug's slim benefits. Karen Weiss, "Efficiency in Drug Development: Knowing the Agency's Expectations to Create a Sound Development Plan," Maximizing Clinical Efficiency Phases conference (Washington, DC, October 9, 2003).

4. Daniel Moerman, *Meaning, Medicine, and the "Placebo Effect"* (Cambridge: Cambridge University Press, 2002), 128.

5. Interview with Robert Temple, 2001.

6. Guy Boulton, "Scientist's Patience Rewarded," *Tampa Tribune*, August 10, 2004, 1.

7. Tim Radford, "Throwing the Microbe into the Bathwater," *The Guardian*, February 22, 1989; Richard Dawood and Jeremy Skidmore, "The Treatment? There Isn't One," *Daily Telegraph*, August 23, 2003, 4; Antiviral Drug Advisory and Research Committee, *Public Hearing NDA 20-871/Nitazoxanide*, transcript, May 6, 1998; interview with Rosemary Soave, January 27, 2005.

8. Antiviral Drug Advisory and Research Committee, *Public Hearing NDA 20-871/Nitazoxanide*, 24.

9. Rosemary Soave, Antiviral Drug Advisory and Research Committee, *Public Hearing NDA 20-871/Nitazoxanide*.

10. O. Doumbo et al., "Nitazoxanide in the Treatment of Cryptosporidial Diarrhea and Other Intestinal Parasitic Infections Associated with Acquired Immunodeficiency Syndrome in Tropical Africa," *American Journal of Tropical Medicine and Hygiene*, June 1997, 637-39.

11. Bob Dudley, Antiviral Drug Advisory and Research Committee, *Public Hearing NDA 20-871/Nitazoxanide*.

12. "AIDS patients sought for study with NTZ for cryptosporidiosis," *Journal of the International Association of Physicians in AIDS Care* 3, no. 6 (June 1997): 48.

13. Antiviral Drug Advisory and Research Committee, *Public Hearing NDA 20-871/Nitazoxanide*.

14. Jon Cohen, *Shots in the Dark: The Wayward Search for an AIDS Vaccine* (New York: W.W. Norton, 2001), 288.

15. Andrew Carr et al., "Treatment of HIV-1-Associated Microsporidiosis and Cryptosporidiosis with Combination Antiretroviral Therapy," *The Lancet*, January 24, 1998, 256-61.

16. Antiviral Drug Advisory and Research Committee, *Public Hearing NDA 20-871/Nitazoxanide*, 158.

17. Ibid.

18. Interview with Rosemary Soave, January 27, 2005.

19. Cynthia Sears, Antiviral Drug Advisory and Research Committee, *Public Hearing NDA 20-871/Nitazoxanide*.

20. Interview with Rosemary Soave, January 27, 2005.

21. Guy Boulton, "Scientist's Patience Rewarded," *Tampa Tribune*, August 10, 2004, 1.

22. Bill Schiller, "Africa's Man of Peace Holds Court in Zambia," *Toronto Star*, August 6, 1989, H1.

23. Lishala C. Situmbeko and Jack Jones Zulu, *Zambia: Condemned to Debt*, World Development Movement, April 2004, 6.

24. Schiller, "Africa's Man of Peace Holds Court in Zambia."

25. Situmbeko and Zulu, *Zambia*, 16-17.

26. Jon Jeter, "Less than $1 Means Family of 6 Can Eat," *Washington Post*, February 19, 2002.

27. Situmbeko and Zulu, *Zambia*, 30.

28. Paul Peachey, "In Foreign Parts: We Could See Many Funerals Here, Warns Mayor as Zambia Stares into the Face of a Devastating Famine," *The Independent*, July 29, 2002.

29. Situmbeko and Zulu, *Zambia*, 30.

30. Sharon LaFraniere, "AIDS Patients in Zambia Face Stark Choices," *New York Times*, October 11, 2003, 1.

31. Mary Gordon, "Fighting AIDS in Zambia," *Toronto Star*, January 18, 2004, F02.

32. Philip J. Hilts, "Out of Africa; Dispelling Myths about AIDS," *Washington Post*, May 24, 1988, Z12.

33. Jonathan Manthorpe, "Kaunda Staring Down Barrel of Democracy," *Ottawa Citizen*, July 28, 1991, F10.

34. Ruth SoRelle, "Seeking an Answer to AIDS," *Houston Chronicle*, April 18, 1993, 10.

35. "Africa's AIDS Pandemic," *Toronto Star*, January 4, 2005, A13.

36. Oakland Ross, "AIDS Pledge 'Opens Floodgates of Hope,' " *Toronto Star*, January 30, 2003, A09.

37. Child Health Research Project, *Synopsis: Persistent Diarrhea Algorithm*, Washington, DC, October 1997.

38. SoRelle, "Seeking an Answer to AIDS."

39. Ibid.

40. Antiviral Drug Advisory and Research Committee, *Public Hearing NDA 20-871/Nitazoxanide*, 26.

41. Interview with Paul S. Kelly, January 26, 2005.

42. SoRelle, "Seeking an Answer to AIDS."

43. Jean-Francois Rossignol et al., "Treatment of Diarrhea Caused by *Cryptosporidium Parvum*: A Prospective, Randomized, Double-Blind, Placebo-Controlled Study of Nitazoxanide," *Journal of Infectious Diseases* 184, no. 1 (2001): 103–6; Jean-Francois Rossignol et al., "Treatment of Diarrhea Caused by *Giardia Intestinalis* and *Entamoegba Histolytica* or *E. Dispar*: A Randomized, Double-Blind, Placebo-Controlled Study of Nitazoxanide," *Journal of Infectious Diseases* 184, no. 3 (2001): 381–84; J. J. Ortiz et al., "Randomized Clinical Study of Nitazoxanide Compared to Metronidazole in the Treatment of Symptomatic Giardiasis in Children from Northern Peru," *Alimentary Pharmacology and Therapeutics* 15 (2001): 1409–15.

44. Paul Kelly et al., "Albendazole Chemotherapy for Treatment of Diarrhoea in Patients with AIDS in Zambia: A Randomised Double Blind Controlled Trial," *BMJ* 312 (1996): 1187–91.

45. The results showed that for HIV-infected children, the drug was no better than placebo. Beatrice Amadi et al., "Effect of Nitazoxanide on Morbidity and Mortality in Zambian Children with Cryptosporidiosis: A Randomized Controlled Trial," *The Lancet*, November 2, 2002, 1375–80.

46. See www.ed.gov/rschstat/research/pubs/rigorousevid/guide_pg5.html.

47. Randomized controlled trials can be conducted with either placebo or "active" controls, and either way they correct for many difficulties in determining the effects of a medical intervention, not least the fact that ordinarily most minor sicknesses and conditions are "self-limiting"; that is, they go away on their own. In addition, chronic problems generally cycle up and down, becoming intense for a while, then lightening up, then becoming intense again. If an experimental drug or new medical intervention is judged solely by how it appears to affect patients, there is no way to account for this. If the patients rally, maybe the drug worked, or perhaps the condition simply improved on its own. Moerman, *Meaning, Medicine, and the "Placebo Effect,"* 12.

48. Mannfred A. Hollinger, *Introduction to Pharmacology* (Philadelphia: Taylor & Francis, 1997), 205.

49. Roy Porter, *The Greatest Benefit to Mankind: A Medical History of Humanity* (New York: W.W. Norton, 1997), 270.

50. Jerry Avorn, *Powerful Medicines: The Benefits, Risks and Costs of Prescription Drugs* (New York: Alfred A. Knopf, 2004), 53.

51. Paul Starr, *The Social Transformation of American Medicine: The Rise of a Sovereign Profession and the Making of a Vast Industry* (New York: Basic Books, 1982), 346; and Sarah Marie Lambert and Howard Markel, "Making History: Thomas Francis, Jr., MD, and the 1954 Salk Poliomyelitis Vaccine Field Trial," *Archives of Pediatrics and Adolescent Medicine*, May 2000, 512.

52. Marcia Meldrum, " 'A Calculated Risk': The Salk Polio Vaccine Field Trials of 1954," *BMJ*, October 31, 1998, 1233–36.

53. Lambert and Markel, "Making History," 512.

54. Anita Guerrini, *Experimenting with Humans and Animals: From Galen to Animal Rights* (Baltimore: Johns Hopkins University Press, 2003), 125; Meldrum, " 'A Calculated Risk.' "

55. While politically palatable, the historical comparison would

certainly dilute the trial's rigor. However the comparison bore out, the results would be open to a range of fair criticism. If fewer vaccinated subjects contracted polio than unvaccinated ones, it could be because they had been less exposed to poliovirus because the weather was different, or perhaps were generally older and could fight off the virus more effectively, or maybe polio in the unvaccinated subjects had been diagnosed differently, and on and on. Since the two groups hadn't been tracked under precisely similar conditions, at the same time, or in the same place, results based on contrasting the groups would be like the proverbial comparison of apples to oranges: no one thing could explain why the two tasted so different. Meldrum, " 'A Calculated Risk.' "

56. Louis Lasagna, "Placebos and Controlled Trials under Attack," *European Journal of Clinical Pharmacology* 15 (1979): 373–74; Pearce Wright, "Louis Lasagna," *The Lancet*, October 25, 2003, 1423; Voice of America, "Science in the News: The Lives of Peter Safar and Louis Lasagna," transcript, August 18, 2003.

57. Robert Temple and Susan S. Ellenberg, "Placebo-Controlled Trials and Active-Control Trials in the Evaluation of New Treatments," *Annals of Internal Medicine*, September 19, 2000, 456–57.

58. E-mail interview with Paul S. Kelly, January 26, 2005.

59. Interview with Rosemary Soave, January 27, 2005.

60. Robert I. Misbin, "Placebo-Controlled Trials in Type 2 Diabetes," *Diabetes Care* 24, no. 4 (2001): 768–74.

61. E-mail correspondence from Joanna Hasegawa, January 25, 2003.

62. E-mail correspondence from Robert Black, January 22, 2005.

63. Most of the infectious diarrhea there stems from viruses, not parasites, with a small percentage caused by bacteria. Rehydration and antibiotics are "the only sensible therapy." E-mail correspondence from Chandra Gulhati, January 25, 2005.

64. R. Rodriguez-Garcia et al., "Effectiveness and Safety of Mebendazole Compared to Nitazoxanide in the Treatment of Giardia Lamblia in Children," *Review Gastroenterology Mexico*, July/September 1999, 122–26; Cesar E. Davila-Gutierrez et al., "Nitazoxanide Compared with Quinfamide and Mebendazole in the Treatment of Helminthic Infections and Intestinal Protozoa in Children," *American Journal of Tropical Medicine and Hygiene* 66,

no. 3 (2002): 251–54; Uri Belkind-Valdovinos, "Evalucion de la nitazoxanida en dosis unica y por tres dias en parasitosis intestinal," *Salud Publica de Mexico*, May/June 2004, 333–40.

65. By February 2005 Kelly was in the process of asking the manufacturers for a quote in order to ascertain whether the University Teaching Hospital might be able to afford a supply of the drug. Interview with Paul S. Kelly, February 16, 2005.

3: Growing the Pharma Monolith

1. Press release, "Salix Pharmaceuticals Announces Positive Results of Rifaximin Study," November 11, 2004.

2. Globalization of Clinical Trials panel, Maximizing Clinical Efficiency Phases conference (Washington, DC, October 9, 2003).

3. Philip J. Hilts, *Protecting America's Health: The FDA, Business, and One Hundred Years of Regulation* (New York: Alfred A. Knopf, 2003), 23–25.

4. Roy Porter, *The Greatest Benefit to Mankind: A Medical History of Humanity* (New York: W.W. Norton, 1997), 368, 663–64.

5. Hilts, *Protecting America's Health*, 46, 53.

6. Paul Ehrlich developed the concept of chemotherapy, synthesizing sulphanilamide in 1907. The drug didn't go into production until after Gerhard Domagk of I.G. Farbenindustrie refined the drug in 1932. Mannfred A. Hollinger, *Introduction to Pharmacology* (Philadelphia: Taylor & Francis, 1997), 207; Porter, *The Greatest Benefit to Mankind*, 452–54.

7. Anita Guerrini, *Experimenting with Humans and Animals: From Galen to Animal Rights* (Baltimore: Johns Hopkins University Press, 2003), 111.

8. Hilts, *Protecting America's Health*, 90; Hollinger, *Introduction to Pharmacology*, 300–301.

9. Back in 1928 a compound produced by a soil mold—penicillin—had been found to have profound bacteria-killing properties. Penicillin didn't just slow bacterial cell growth, as sulfanilamide did—it killed the cells outright. Not only that, the compound attacked bacterial cells selectively, leaving mammalian

cells untouched and making even large doses of the drug theoretically safe for humans. The trouble was that the mold produced vanishingly small amounts of the compound, and even these quantities deteriorated fast. Producing enough stable penicillin to treat a single patient had proven so difficult for researchers at Oxford that they had resorted to recycling the chemical from the patient's urine; in the end, the team ran out of penicillin and the infected patient had perished. Hollinger, *Introduction to Pharmacology*, 134–35; Porter, *The Greatest Benefit to Mankind*, 456–57; Hilts, *Protecting America's Health*, 101–4.

10. Laurie Garrett, *Betrayal of Trust: The Collapse of Global Public Health* (New York: Hyperion, 2000), 323.

11. Ironically, at the time leading drug companies all refused to develop this promising drug into a more practical one, despite the entreaties of government officials. They considered the investment too risky, worrying that the life-saving drug might suddenly stop working, as had happened with sulfa drugs. Only after a government-sponsored project figured out how to increase the mold's yield of the drug by 120-fold did drug companies reluctantly agree to start producing penicillin. Hilts, *Protecting America's Health*, 102–3.

12. Paul Starr, *The Social Transformation of American Medicine: The Rise of a Sovereign Profession and the Making of a Vast Industry* (New York: Basic Books, 1982), 342.

13. "Funding for Health Research and Development, According to Source of Funds: United States, Selected Fiscal Years 1970–99," in *Health, United States, 2001* (Hyattsville, MD: National Center for Health Statistics, 2001), 346.

14. Fran Hawthorne, *The Merck Druggernaut: The Inside Story of a Pharmaceutical Giant* (Hoboken, NJ: John Wiley & Sons, 2003), 26.

15. Daniel Callahan, *What Price Better Health? Hazards of the Research Imperative* (Los Angeles: University of California Press, 2003), 237.

16. Hilts, *Protecting America's Health*, 121–22, 130.

17. Ibid., 146–47.

18. Jordan Goodman, Anthony McElligot, and Lara Marks, eds., *Useful Bodies: Humans in the Service of Medical Science in the Twentieth Century* (Baltimore: Johns Hopkins University, 2003), 14.

19. Hollinger, *Introduction to Pharmacology*, 92, 109; Hilts, *Protecting America's Health*, 150.

20. Hilts, *Protecting America's Health*, 149.

21. Ibid., 144–54.

22. The condition had previously been so rare that few physicians had ever seen it before. Medical editors rushed to find photographs to illustrate the condition in their new textbooks but came up empty-handed. They resorted to Francisco de Goya's nineteenth-century painting of a phocomelic infant instead. Hollinger, *Introduction to Pharmacology*, 108.

23. Hilts, *Protecting America's Health*, 155.

24. Ibid., 131–43, 157–58.

25. Ibid., 164.

26. Hollinger, *Introduction to Pharmacology*, 310.

27. Allen A. Mitchell, "Systematic Identification of Drugs That Cause Birth Defects—a New Opportunity," *New England Journal of Medicine*, December 25, 2003, 2556–59.

28. Instead, the new rules required proof of efficacy, even though whether thalidomide worked was never really the issue. Just a few years after its fall from grace, thalidomide was resurrected as a treatment for leprosy. The drug continued to be used by pregnant women, who predictably bore phocomelic babies, particularly in Portuguese-speaking Brazil, where thalidomide was sold with English-language warnings on the side of the box. A drug with complex clinical effects, thalidomide is currently being investigated as a treatment for a range of diseases, from cancers to AIDS. Now sedation is considered the "side" effect. Vittal Katikireddi, "Thalidomide: A Second Chance?" *BMJ*, February 14, 2004, 412; "Thalidomide: A Second Chance?" BBC program transcript, February 12, 2004, available at www.bbc.co.uk/science/horizon/2004/thalidomidetrans.shtml.

29. Hilts, *Protecting America's Health*, 161, 164–65, 172.

30. Sandra Panem, *The Interferon Crusade* (Washington, DC: Brookings Institution, 1984), 2.

31. See, for example, web.mit.edu/invent/a-winners/a-boyer cohen.html.

32. See, for example, www.amgen.com/rnd/history.html.

33. Hawthorne, *The Merck Druggernaut*, 24.

34. Panem, *The Interferon Crusade*, 86.

35. Hilts, *Protecting America's Health*, 255.

36. "Percentage of New Products and Processes That Were Dependent on Academic Research, for Selected Industries in the United States: 1975–85," *Science and Engineering Indicators, 2000* (Arlington, VA: National Science Foundation, 2000), 7–18.

37. U.S. Bureau of Census, "National Health Expenditures—Summary, 1960 to 1999, and projections, 2000 to 2010," *Statistical Abstract of the U.S.: 2001*, Washington, DC, January 2002, 91. The economy as a whole, in contrast, just bettered doubling in size. The GDP in 1974 was $1,635.2 billion; the GDP in 1984 was $3,932.7 billion. "Population and U.S. Gross Domestic Product, 1949–2000," *Annual Energy Review, 2000* (Washington, DC: Energy Information Administration, August 2001), 351.

38. Martha M. Hamilton, "Drug Companies Lobby to Revise Compromise Bill," *Washington Post*, July 29, 1984, G1.

39. Katherine Greider, *The Big Fix: How the Pharmaceutical Industry Rips Off American Consumers* (New York: PublicAffairs, 2003), 30–31.

40. See "Drop in Death Rates for Diseases Treated with Pharmaceuticals, 1965–1996," available at www.quintiles.com, citing U.S. National Center for Health Statistics 1998.

41. Porter, *The Greatest Benefit to Mankind*, 718.

42. Hawthorne, *The Merck Druggernaut*, 85.

43. Garrett, *Betrayal of Trust*, 374.

44. Joe Graedon and Teresa Greadon, "On the Horizon: New Drugs Show Promise," *St. Louis Dispatch*, January 2, 1990, 8D.

45. Sally Squires, "Even Young Adults Can Increase Life Expectancy by Cutting Cholesterol," *Washington Post*, December 11, 1985, 5.

46. Morton Mintz, "Critics Sound Alarm as Firms Pin Hopes on Cholesterol Drug," *Washington Post*, March 8, 1987, H5.

47. Hilts, *Protecting America's Health*, 144–45.

48. Maryann Napoli, "Cholesterol Skeptics and the Bad News about Statin Drugs," Center for Medical Consumers, June 2003, available at www.medicalconsumers.org/pages/cholesterol_skeptics.html.

49. Mevacor was followed by the release of Prozac in 1987. The market for drugs to treat depression wasn't a very big one at the time. Before 1980, depression was considered a relatively rare

condition, treated primarily with psychotherapy or tranquilizers. Psychiatrists also prescribed the so-called tricyclic drugs, cheap meds that had been developed in the 1950s. In the early 1980s, Astra and Duphar Laboratories had tried and failed to cut into the depression market with "selective serotonin reuptake inhibitors" (SSRI) drugs like Prozac, which tinkered with serotonin levels in the brain. But SSRI drugs Zelmid and Luvox didn't work any better than the tricyclic antidepressants, had unexpected and unacceptable side effects, and were more expensive to boot. The drugs bombed.

Eli Lilly didn't bother proving that Prozac was more effective than the other SSRIs or the older tricyclic antidepressants. The drug barely worked better than placebo. In four of the eight centers that conducted placebo-controlled trials of Prozac for the drug's FDA application, patients improved more on placebos than Prozac. But the FDA approved the drug regardless. After all, Prozac didn't need to be more effective than already available antidepressants. According to drugmaker Eli Lilly, Prozac was safer. To their physicians' chagrin, some depressed patients on tricyclic drugs crossed the thin line dividing medicine from poison, using their antidepressants as toxins with which to kill themselves. Such patients would remain just as depressed and suicidal on Prozac, but they wouldn't be able to use the drug for this purpose, as it is nearly impossible to die from an overdose of Prozac. The drug also appeared to be more acceptable to patients—fewer dropped out of trials because of irritating side effects such as constipation and dry mouth.

The lack of pesky side effects and its one-size-fits-all dosing made Prozac "an easy drug for doctors to prescribe," London's *Independent* noted. It was just in the nick of time. Employers were "wary of paying the bill for a lifetime of 45-minute sessions for long-winded Woody Allens," as *Forbes* put it. If eons of expensive talk therapy could be eliminated with ten-second scribbles on a prescription pad, so be it.

Within a year of its release, Prozac was the bestselling antidepressant drug of all time. In 1989, about six million Americans took home prescriptions for the new drug, more than double the number who had popped the just as effective but much cheaper tricyclic drugs less than a decade before. Sufferers banded together with Lilly to "raise awareness" about the scourge of depression. Some patient groups conveniently shared offices with the PR offices of drug companies selling the spanking new antidepressants.

Whereas depression had once been considered rare, now it was considered all too common, afflicting no fewer than one in ten Americans, more of whom now sought help, which more often came in the form of Prozac or another of the SSRI drugs that followed hot on Prozac's trail. Magazines splashed Prozac on their covers, dubbing it a "wonder drug" and a "breakthrough." Even pet dogs were put on Prozac. David Healy, *Let Them Eat Prozac: The Unhealthy Relationship Between the Pharmaceutical Industry and Depression* (New York: New York University Press, 2004), 35, 111; M.S. Lima and J. Moncrieff, "Drugs Versus Placebo for Dysthymia (Cochrane Review)," in *The Cochrane Library*, issue 3 (Chichester, UK: John Wiley & Sons, 2004); Richard Grant, "The Prozac Generation," *The Independent*, January 30, 1994, 12; Robert Langreth, "Just Say No," *Forbes.com*, November 29, 2004; Natalie Angier, "New Antidepressant Is Acclaimed but Not Perfect," *New York Times*, March 29, 1990, 9; Paul E. Greenberg et al., "The Economic Burden of Depression in the United States: How Did It Change Between 1990 and 2000?" *Journal of Clinical Psychiatry*, December 2003, 1465–73.

50. Hawthorne, *The Merck Druggernaut*, 37.

51. Ranjit B. Mani, "The Evaluation of Disease Modifying Therapies in Alzheimer's Disease: A Regulatory Viewpoint," *Statistics in Medicine* 23 (2004): 305–14.

52. J.A. O'Shaughnessy et al., "Commentary Concerning Demonstration of Safety and Efficacy of Investigational Anticancer Agents in Clinical Trials," *Journal of Clinical Oncology*, December 1991, 2225–32.

53. Thomas R. Fleming and David L. DeMets, "Surrogate End Points in Clinical Trials: Are We Being Misled?" *Annals of Internal Medicine*, October 1, 1996, 605; see also Bruce M. Psaty et al., "Surrogate End Points, Health Outcomes, and the Drug-Approval Process for the Treatment of Risk Factors for Cardiovascular Disease," *JAMA*, August 25, 1999, 786–90.

54. Cardiologists had been so certain of the drugs' lifesaving abilities—touted by magazines such as *U.S. News & World Report*—that when the placebo-controlled trial was first proposed

at a meeting, some were moved to cry "You are immoral! You are immoral!" from the audience. Hilts, *Protecting America's Health*, 231; Associated Press, "Researcher Links Heart Drugs to 2,250 Deaths," *New York Times*, July 26, 1989, 13.

55. Fleming and DeMets, "Surrogate End Points in Clinical Trials."

56. Food and Drug Administration, "Establishment of Prescription Drug User Fee Rates for Fiscal Year 2005," *Federal Register*, August 2, 2004; Greider, *The Big Fix*, 105.

57. Hilts, *Protecting America's Health*, 336.

58. Greider, *The Big Fix*, 105.

59. Washington Business Information/FDAnews, "Senate Bill to Give FDA Authority over Tobacco Products Finds Unlikely Support," June 4, 2004.

60. Editorial, "The Hazards of Seldane," *New York Times*, January 17, 1997, 30.

61. John Schwartz, "FDA Relaxes Rules for On-Air Drug Ads; Changes Allow Product's Purpose to Be Stated," *Washington Post*, August 9, 1997, 1.

62. Ibid.

63. Milt Freudenheim, "Influencing Doctor's Orders," *New York Times*, November 17, 1998, 2.

64. Ibid.

65. Francesca Lunzer Kritz, "Ask Your Doctor About . . . ," *Washington Post*, June 6, 2000, Z09.

66. J. Van Steekelenburg et al., "Comparison of Five New Antihistamines (H1-Receptor Antagonists) in Patients with Allergic Rhinitis Using Nasal Provocation Studies and Skin Tests," *Allergy* 57 (2002): 346–50.

67. Schwartz, "FDA Relaxes Rules for On-Air Drug Ads."

68. Freudenheim, "Influencing Doctor's Orders."

69. Gina Kolata, "U.S. Approves Sales of Impotence Pill; Huge Market Seen," *New York Times*, March 28, 1998.

70. Henry A. Feldman et al., "Erectile Dysfunction and Coronary Risk Factors: Prospective Results from the Massachusetts Male Aging Study," *Preventive Medicine* 30 (2000): 328–38.

71. Carol A. Derby et al., "Modifiable Risk Factors and Erectile Dysfunction: Can Lifestyle Changes Modify Risk?" *Urology*, August 2000, 302–6.

72. David Tuller, "Gentlemen, Start Your Engines?" *New York Times*, June 21, 2004, F1.

73. Peter Carlson, "Potent Medicine: A Year Ago, Viagra Hit the Shelves and the Earth Moved. Well, Sort Of," *Washington Post*, March 26, 1999, C1.

74. Greider, *The Big Fix*, 118.

75. Tuller, "Gentlemen, Start Your Engines?"

76. Ibid.

77. "Viagra Swells Diagnosis Rates for Erectile Dysfunction," *BMJ*, February 2003, 326.

78. Carlson, "Potent Medicine."

79. Claude Lenfant, "Clinical Research to Clinical Practice—Lost in Translation?" *New England Journal of Medicine*, August 28, 2003, 868–74.

80. Carlson, "Potent Medicine."

81. Judith Aldridge and Fiona Measham, "Sildenafil (Viagra) Is Used as a Recreational Drug in England," *BMJ*, March 1999, 669.

82. Carlson, "Potent Medicine."

83. Knight-Ridder, "Double Your Pleasure, Double Your Fun . . . ," *Toronto Star*, June 14, 2003, C11.

84. Jay S. Cohen, *Overdose: The Case Against the Drug Companies* (New York: Jeremy P. Tarcher/Putnam, 2001), 51.

85. "The Lifestyle Drugs Outlook to 2005," Executive Summary, Reuters Business Insight, February 1999, reprinted at www.inpharm.com/intelligence/rbi080299.html; "The Lifestyle Drugs Outlook to 2008: Unlocking New Value in Well-Being," Summary, Reuters Business Insight, October 2003, at www.the-infoshop.com/study/rb16175_lifestyle_drugs.html.

86. Paul Abrahams, "Taking Health to Heart—How Much Cholesterol Is Too Much?" *Financial Times*, October 23, 1992, 18.

87. Marcia Angell, *The Truth about the Drug Companies: How They Deceive Us and What to Do about It* (New York: Random House, 2004), 54.

88. Hawthorne, *The Merck Druggernaut*, 69.

89. Jun Ma et al., "A Statistical Analysis of the Magnitude and Composition of Drug Promotion in the United States in 1998," *Clinical Therapeutics*, May 2003, 1503–17.

90. Angell, *The Truth about the Drug Companies*, 133.

91. National Institute for Health Care Management Foundation, *Prescription Drug Expenditures in 2001: Another Year of Escalating Costs*, Washington, DC, May 6, 2002, 13; editorial, "The Statin Wars: Why AstraZeneca Must Retreat," *The Lancet*, October 25, 2003.

92. Jeffrey J. Ellis et al., "Suboptimal Statin Adherence and Discontinuation in Primary and Secondary Prevention Populations," *Journal of General Internal Medicine*, June 2004, 638.

93. Napoli, "Cholesterol Skeptics and the Bad News about Statin Drugs."

94. Jonathan D. Quick et al., "Ensuring Ethical Drug Promotion—Whose Responsibility?" *The Lancet*, August 30, 2003.

95. Editorial, "The Statin Wars."

96. Stephen S. Hall, "The Claritin Effect: Prescription for Profit," *New York Times Magazine*, March 11, 2001, 40.

97. Cohen, *Overdose*, 92.

98. At least thirty-one cases of fatal rhabdomyolysis attributed to Baycol were reported to the FDA. According to the FDA, reports of adverse drug reactions constitute about 5 percent of the actual number of reactions. Ibid., 5.

99. Public Citizen press release, "Cases of Kidney Failure, Muscle Damage Should Prompt FDA to Ban Crestor," *Worst Pills, Best Pills*, Washington, DC, March 4, 2004. The FDA rejected Public Citizen's request that it ban the drug.

100. Cohen, *Overdose*, 148.

101. Craig G. Burkhart et al., "The *Physicians' Desk Reference* Should Not Be Held as a Legal Standard of Medical Care," *Archives of Pediatric and Adolescent Medicine*, June 1998, 609–10.

102. Cohen, *Overdose*, 149–50.

103. Joseph S. Ross et al., *Medical Education Services Suppliers: A Threat to Physician Education*, Public Citizen Health Research Group, Washington, DC, July 19, 2000.

104. "Myocardial Infarction: State-Required CME: No Effect on Heart Attack Care, Boosts Use of Branded Drugs," *Heart Disease Weekly*, April 4, 2004, 89.

105. David A. Kessler et al., "Therapeutic-Class Wars—Drug Promotion in a Competitive Marketplace," *New England Journal of Medicine*, November 17, 1994, 1350–53.

106. National Institute for Health Care Management Foundation, *Prescription Drug Expenditures in 2001*, 3.

107. NIH Director's Panel on Clinical Research, *Report to the Advisory Committee to the NIH Director*, Executive Summary, December 1997, available at www.nih.gov/news/crp/97report/execsum.htm.

108. "Funding for Health Research and Development, According to Source of Funds: United States, Selected Fiscal Years 1970–99," in *Health, United States, 2001*, 346.

109. Scott Hensley, "Remedial Lessons: When Doctors Go to Class, Industry Often Foots the Bill," *Wall Street Journal*, December 4, 2002, A1.

110. Marcia Angell, "Is Academic Medicine for Sale?" *New England Journal of Medicine*, May 18, 2000, 1516–18.

111. Peter Jaret, "She Turns Her Pen on Drug Makers," *Los Angeles Times*, August 9, 2004.

112. Jerry Avorn, *Powerful Medicines: The Benefits, Risks, and Costs of Prescription Drugs* (New York: Alfred A. Knopf, 2004), 53.

113. Plus, patient response to drugs can be colored by all sorts of underlying factors besides the drug's pharmacologic mechanism, especially in short trials of poorly understood conditions. In one study of anxiety green pills worked better than pills of other colors, even though they had the same medicine in them; in a study of depression, yellow pills worked better than pills of other colors. Researchers can relieve pain in patients simply by telling them they are receiving an effective painkiller, even while giving them placebos instead. For some conditions no fewer than 30 percent of patients in clinical trials improve on placebos alone. Not only that: injected placebos work better than pills, and two placebos work better than one. In all of these studies placebos work only if the patients know they are getting some treatment; if the placebos are surreptitiously dropped into drinks or IV lines, they have no effect. In other words, "it is not the placebo itself . . . it is the knowledge of the placebo that does the trick." Daniel Moerman, *Meaning, Medicine, and the "Placebo Effect"* (Cambridge: Cambridge University Press, 2002), 49, 105–6. See also Thomas Bodenheimer, "Uneasy Alliance—Clinical Investigators and the Pharmaceutical Industry," *New England Journal of Medicine*, May 18, 2000, 1539–44.

114. Bodenheimer, "Uneasy Alliance."

115. See depts.washington.edu/gim/faculty/psaty.htm

116. Gina Kolata, "Blood Pressure Drug Linked to Heart Risks," *Houston Chronicle*, March 12, 1995, 4.

117. Warren King, "Risk Cited for Blood Pressure Drug—Chances Higher for Heart Attack," *Seattle Times*, March 10, 1995.

118. "Controlling Your High Blood Pressure; Reports Cause Furor by Linking Some Drugs to Heart Attack Risk," *Washington Post*, March 28, 1995, Z10.

119. Harry Schwartz, "The Great Calcium Channel Blocker Scare," *Pharmaceutical Executive*, June 1994, 24.

120. R.A. Deyo et al., "The Messenger under Attack—Intimidation of Researchers by Special-Interest Groups," *New England Journal of Medicine*, April 17, 1997, 1176–80.

121. National Institute for Health Care Management Foundation, *Prescription Drug Expenditures in 2001*, 2; Greider, *The Big Fix*, 3.

122. Greider, *The Big Fix*.

123. Interview with Mark McClellan, October 9, 2003.

124. James S. Gordon, "The Risk of Taking the Right Drugs," *Washington Post*, August 17, 2003, citing *Archives of Internal Medicine* studies.

125. Hilts, *Protecting America's Health*, 307.

126. Cohen, *Overdose*, 4.

127. Greider, *The Big Fix*, 131.

128. National Institutes of Health, *Guidelines for the Conduct of Research Involving Human Subjects at the National Institutes of Health*, August 2004.

4: Uncaging the Guinea Pig

1. Roy Porter, *The Greatest Benefit to Mankind: A Medical History of Humanity* (New York: W.W. Norton, 1997), 38, 57–59, 138, 153.

2. Anita Guerrini, *Experimenting with Humans and Animals: From Galen to Animal Rights* (Baltimore: Johns Hopkins University Press, 2003); Porter, *The Greatest Benefit to Mankind*, 23, 67, 76, 132, 182.

3. Guerrini, *Experimenting with Humans and Animals*, 86.

4. Susan M. Reverby, ed., *Tuskegee's Truths: Rethinking the Tuskegee Syphilis Study* (Chapel Hill: University of North Carolina

Press, 2000), 19; Porter, *The Greatest Benefit to Mankind*, 166–67, 175, 190.

5. Reverby, ed., *Tuskegee's Truths*, 67.

6. Laurie Garrett, *Betrayal of Trust: The Collapse of Global Public Health* (New York: Hyperion, 2000), 321; Reverby, ed., *Tuskegee's Truths*, 367.

7. Margaret Humphreys, "Whose Body? Which Disease?" in Jordan Goodman, Anthony McElligot, and Lara Marks, eds., *Useful Bodies: Humans in the Service of Medical Science in the Twentieth Century* (Baltimore: Johns Hopkins University Press, 2003), 55, 64–69; Reverby, ed., *Tuskegee's Truths*, 300.

8. Reverby, ed., *Tuskegee's Truths*, 18, 80, 368.

9. Ibid., 269–72.

10. Ibid., 22–25.

11. Ibid., 28, 126.

12. Ibid., 15, 25; Guerrini, *Experimenting with Humans and Animals*, 109.

13. But penicillin, it seemed, was too good to pass up. Almost a third of the Tuskegee subjects managed, somehow, to get a few doses of the drug; around 7 percent received therapeutically adequate doses. The results from the trial were thus compromised. Reverby, ed., *Tuskegee's Truths*, 26.

14. Jonathan D. Moreno, *Undue Risk: Secret State Experiments on Humans* (New York: W.H. Freeman, 2000), 29–31, 33–34, 66.

15. Ibid., 36–37.

16. Ibid., 215–18.

17. David S. Jones and Robert L. Martensen, "Human Radiation Experiments and the Formation of Medical Physics at the University of California, San Francisco and Berkeley, 1937–1962," in Goodman, McElligot, and Marks, eds., *Useful Bodies*, 97.

18. Moreno, *Undue Risk*, 122–229.

19. Ibid., 50.

20. Daniel Callahan, *What Price Better Health? Hazards of the Research Imperative* (Los Angeles: University of California Press, 2003), 138.

21. Moreno, *Undue Risk*, 98.

22. Ibid., 72.

23. Ibid., 57.

24. Jones and Martensen, "Human Radiation Experiments," 86.

25. Guerrini, *Experimenting with Humans and Animals*, 138.

26. Moreno, *Undue Risk*, 68.

27. Reverby, ed., *Tuskegee's Truths*, 25.

28. Moreno, *Undue Risk*, 77.

29. Moreno, *Undue Risk*, 55; Porter, *The Greatest Benefit to Mankind*, 649.

30. Moreno, *Undue Risk*, 75.

31. *Trials of War Criminals before the Nuremberg Military Tribunals under Control Council Law* 2, no. 10 (1949): 181–82, available at ohsr.od.nih.gov/guidelines/nuremberg.html.

32. Moreno, *Undue Risk*, 80.

33. How much did good science depend upon good ethics, anyway? After the war U.S. officials actively recruited thousands of the best and brightest German scientists and engineers to work in American government agencies—including those who had been involved in Nazi medical experiments. Moreno, *Undue Risk*, 92–93, 101, 130; Advisory Committee on Human Radiation Experiments, "History of Prison Research Regulation," *Final Report*, at tis.eh.doe.gov/ohre/roadmap/achre/chap9_4.html.

34. Guerrini, *Experimenting with Humans and Animals*, 123–28.

35. Moreno, *Undue Risk*, 132–33, 154.

36. Joel D. Howell and Rodney A. Hayward, "Writing Willowbrook, Reading Willowbrook," in Goodman, McElligot, and Marks, eds., *Useful Bodies*, 193.

37. Reporter Geraldo Rivera exposed the appalling conditions at Willowbrook in a 1972 television program, ultimately leading to a class-action lawsuit. Shaila K. Dewan, "Recalling a Victory for the Disabled," *New York Times*, May 3, 2000, 5; Margaret Engel, "Care for the Mentally Retarded: A Case History," *Washington Post*, December 30, 1984.

38. Merck later capitalized on Krugman's work by developing a hepatitis B vaccine, which they tested on their own executives. In a wry comment on Krugman's trials a Merck scientist joked in 1975 that the company had "picked the most worthless people we could find in the world who would be the least likely to sue." If Merck hadn't, Krugman certainly had. Jon Cohen, *Shots in the Dark: The Wayward Search for an AIDS Vaccine* (New York: W.W. Norton, 2001), 79; David J. Rothman, *Strangers at the Bedside:*

A History of How Law and Bioethics Transformed Medical Decision Making (New York: Basic Books, 1991), 77.

39. Guerrini, *Experimenting with Humans and Animals*, 139, citing Henry Beecher, "Ethics and Clinical Research," *New England Journal of Medicine* 264 (1966): 1354–60; Howell and Hayward, "Writing Willowbrook, Reading Willowbrook," 192.

40. Reverby, ed., *Tuskegee's Truths*, 103.

41. Elizabeth W. Etheridge, "Historical Perspectives: History of CDC," *Morbidity and Mortality Weekly Report*, June 28, 1996, 526–30, at www.cdc.gov/epo/mmwr/preview/mmwrhtml/00042732.htm.

42. Reverby, ed., *Tuskegee's Truths*, 15, 26, 411.

43. Ibid., 152–54.

44. U.S. Bureau of Census, "National Health Expenditures—Summary, 1960 to 1999, and Projections, 2000 to 2010," *Statistical Abstract of the U.S.: 2001*, Washington, DC, January 2002, 91.

45. Paul Starr, *The Social Transformation of American Medicine: The Rise of a Sovereign Profession and the Making of a Vast Industry* (New York: Basic Books, 1982), 381–82, 409, citing "It's Time to Operate," *Fortune*, January 1970, 79, and Ivan Illich, *Medical Nemesis: The Expropriation of Health* (New York: Pantheon, 1976).

46. Some sections of the medical community, however, were not nearly so provoked. An editorial in the October 1972 issue of the *Southern Medical Journal* condemned the "irresponsible press": "In complete disregard of their abysmal ignorance, members of the fourth estate bang out anything on their typewriters which will make headlines," the editorial fumed. "If the men having latent syphilis . . . had been *forced* to take adequate treatment (60 or more weekly doses of a metal [mercury]), cardiovascular syphilis might have been avoided in most. In our free society, antisyphilitic treatment has never been forced. Since these men did not elect to obtain treatment available to them, the development of aortic disease lay at the subject's door and not in the Study's protocol." Reverby, ed., *Tuskegee's Truths*, 2, 177, 199; Vernal G. Cave, "Proper Uses and Abuses of the Health Care Delivery System for Minorities, with Special Reference to the Tuskegee Syphilis Study," *Journal of the National Medical Association* 67 (1975), reprinted in Reverby, ed., *Tuskegee's Truths*, 399.

47. Reverby, ed., *Tuskegee's Truths*, 229; Garrett, *Betrayal of Trust*, 322

48. Guerrini, *Experimenting with Humans and Animals*, 141–47.

49. World Medical Association, "Declaration of Helsinki: Ethical Principles for Medical Research Involving Human Subjects," available at www.wma.net.

50. U.S. Food and Drug Administration, *Guidance for Industry: Acceptance of Foreign Clinical Studies*, March 2001; also *Code of Federal Regulations Title 21*, vol. 5, April 2005, 21CFR312.120; National Institutes of Health, *Guidelines for the Conduct of Research Involving Human Subjects*, August 2001.

5: HIV and the Second-rate Solution

1. World Medical Association, "Declaration of Helsinki: Ethical Principles for Medical Research Involving Human Subjects," available at www.wma.net.

2. Laurie Garrett, *The Coming Plague: Newly Emerging Diseases in a World Out of Balance* (New York: Penguin Books, 1994), 302.

3. Philip J. Hilts, *Protecting America's Health: The FDA, Business, and One Hundred Years of Regulation* (New York: Alfred A. Knopf, 2003), 242.

4. "As a profession, we doctors are not only determined, but also somewhat obsessed with primacy," one commentator later noted, drily. "To the victors belongs more than mere mention in a medical textbook; discovering something first may be a medical investigator's best shot at immortality." Howard Markel, " 'Who's on First?'—Medical Discoveries and Scientific Priority," *New England Journal of Medicine*, December 30, 2004, 2792–93. See also Jon Cohen, *Shots in the Dark: The Wayward Search for an AIDS Vaccine* (New York: W.W. Norton, 2001), 18.

5. Cohen, *Shots in the Dark*, 41.

6. Mark Simpson, "Angry with a Capital A," *The Guardian*, June 19, 1995, T42.

7. Barnaby J. Feder, "Drug Expected to Spur Growth and Profit of Its Maker," *Washington Post*, September 6, 1988; editorial, "AZT's Inhuman Cost," *New York Times*, August 28, 1989, 16.

8. Interview with Jay Brooks Jackson, October 10, 2003.

9. Susan Okie, "Testing of New AIDS Drugs Beset by Conflicting Demands," *Washington Post*, September 6, 1988.

10. Richard Lynn and G. Harold Mehlman, "Why ACT UP Did What It Did," *Washington Post*, June 2, 1990, A17.

11. Okie, "Testing of New AIDS Drugs Beset by Conflicting Demands."

12. Jay Brooks Jackson et al., "HIVNET 012: A Phase III Placebo-Controlled Trial to Determine the Efficacy of Oral AZT and the Efficacy of Oral Nevirapine for the Prevention of Vertical Transmission of HIV-1 Infection in Pregnant Ugandan Women and Their Neonates," National Institute of Allergy and Infectious Disease IND#49,991 study protocol, June 5, 1997.

13. Peter Lurie and Sidney Wolfe, "Unethical Trials of Interventions to Reduce Perinatal Transmission of the Human Immunodeficiency Virus in Developing Countries," *New England Journal of Medicine*, September 18, 1997.

14. Interview with Peter Lurie, October 9, 2003.

15. U.S. Public Health Service Task Force on the Use of Zidovudine to Reduce Perinatal HIV Transmission, "Recommendations of the U.S. Public Health Service Task Force on the Use of Zidovudine to Reduce Perinatal Human Immunodeficiency Virus," *Morbidity and Mortality Weekly Report*, August 5, 1994, 1–20.

16. See www.fda.gov/ohrms/dockets/ac/03/transcripts/3932T1.htm.

17. See www.fda.gov/oashi/aids/miles91.html.

18. Viramune (nevirapine) patient information, available at www.viramune.com/PatientInfo/.

19. Brian Vastag, "Helsinki Discord? A Controversial Declaration," *JAMA*, December 20, 2000, 2984.

20. Donald G. McNeil, "Africans Outdo U.S. Patients in Following AIDS Therapy," *New York Times*, September 3, 2003, 1.

21. Ibid.

22. Ira Flatow, "Talk of the Nation Science Friday: Medical Ethics, School Computers," National Public Radio transcript, September 26, 1997.

23. Elliot Marseille et al., "Cost Effectiveness of Single-Dose Nevirapine Regimen for Mothers and Babies to Decrease Vertical HIV-1 Transmission in Sub-Saharan Africa," *The Lancet*,

September 4, 1999; letter from Neal Halsey to Harold Varmus, May 6, 1997.

24. World Health Organization, "Recommendations from the Meeting on Mother-to-Infant Transmission of HIV by Use of Anti-retrovirals," Geneva, June 23–25, 1994; letter from Neal Halsey to Harold Varmus, May 6, 1997; Sheryl Gay Stolberg, "Placebo Use Is Suspended in Overseas AIDS Trials," *New York Times*, February 19, 1998, 16.

25. Peter Lurie et al., "Ethical, Behavioral, and Social Aspects of HIV Vaccine Trials in Developing Countries," *JAMA*, January 26, 1994.

26. Interview with Peter Lurie, October 9, 2003.

27. Cohen, *Shots in the Dark*, 248.

28. Ibid., 243, 161–65.

29. Ibid., 261, 268–69.

30. Ibid., 266.

31. Ibid., 69.

32. Peter Wehrwein and Kelly Morris, "HIV-1-Vaccine-Trial Go-Ahead Reawakens Ethics Debate," *The Lancet*, June 13, 1998, 1789.

33. Interview with Jay Brooks Jackson, October 10, 2003; Anne Bennett Swingle, "The Pathologist Who Struck Gold," *Hopkins Medical News*, Spring/Summer 2001.

34. Swingle, "The Pathologist Who Struck Gold."

35. Brooks Jackson et al., "HIVNET 012."

36. Ibid.

37. Interview with Jay Brooks Jackson, October 10, 2003.

38. Stefan Z. Wiktor et al., "Short-Course Oral Zidovudine for Prevention of Mother-to-Child Transmission of HIV-1 in Abidjan, Cote d'Ivoire: A Randomized Trial," *The Lancet*, March 6, 1999, 781–85; Nathan Shaffer et al., "Short-Course Zidovudine for Perinatal HIV-1 Transmission in Bangkok, Thailand: A Randomized Controlled Trial," *The Lancet*, March 6, 1999, 773.

39. Catherine Wilfert et al., "Science, Ethics, and Future of Research into Maternal Infant Transmission of HIV-1," *The Lancet*, March 6, 1999, 832.

40. Interview with Peter Lurie, October 8, 2003.

41. Esther Iverem, "The Silent Treatment," *Washington Post*, February 22, 1997, H1.

42. Interview with Peter Lurie, October 8, 2003.

43. Lurie and Wolfe, "Unethical Trials of Interventions," 853–56.

44. Marcia Angell, "The Ethics of Clinical Research in the Third World," *New England Journal of Medicine*, September 18, 1997, 847–49; Sheryl Gay Stolberg, "U.S. AIDS Research Abroad Sets Off Outcry over Ethics," *New York Times*, September 18, 1997, A1.

45. Jonathan Bor, "Editorial Writer Heard 'Round Medical World," *Baltimore Sun*, October 26, 1997.

46. Correspondence from Neal A. Holtzman to Sidney Wolfe, October 14, 1997.

47. Flatow, "Talk of the Nation Science Friday."

48. Interview with Jonathan D. Moreno, March 21, 2005.

49. Neal Halsey et al., "Ethics and International Research: Research Standards Are the Same Throughout the World; Medical Care Is Not," *BMJ*, October 18, 1997.

50. Wilfert et al., "Science, Ethics, and Future of Research," 832–35.

51. Shaffer et al., "Short-Course Zidovudine," 773–79; Wiktor et al., "Short-Course Oral Zidovudine."

52. Jonathan Bor, "Ethics of AIDS Trials Is Debated," *Baltimore Sun*, September 18, 1997.

53. Wilfert et al., "Science, Ethics, and Future of Research," 832–35.

54. UNAIDS, "Ethical Considerations in HIV Preventive Vaccine Research, guidance document, May 2000, cited in World Medical Association, "Workgroup Report on the Revision of Paragraph 30 of the Declaration of Helsinki," September 2003.

55. Lurie joined Sidney Wolfe at Public Citizen. Marcia Angell was forced out of the editor's chair at the *New England Journal of Medicine* in 2000, amid "heated disagreements" over commercializing the journal. Michele Kurtz, "A Guiding Light at the New England Journal," *Boston Globe*, July 6, 2004, D8.

56. Cohen, *Shots in the Dark*, 276, 286, 348–49

57. Ibid., 354.

58. Interview with Peter Lurie, October 2003.

59. Interview with Jay Brooks Jackson, October 10, 2003.

60. Swingle, "The Pathologist Who Struck Gold."

61. Johns Hopkins Medical Institutions Office of Communications and Public Affairs press release, "Brooks Jackson Named New Director of Hopkins Pathology," September 28, 2001.

62. Marc Lallemant et al., correspondence, "Ethics of Placebo-Controlled Trials of Zidovudine to Prevent the Perinatal Transmission of HIV in the Third World," *New England Journal of Medicine*, March 19, 1998; Marc Lallemant et al., "A Trial of Shortened Zidovudine Regimens to Prevent Mother-to-Child Transmission of Human Immunodeficiency Virus Type 1," *New England Journal of Medicine*, October 5, 2000.

63. Elliot Marseille et al., "Cost Effectiveness of Single-Dose Nevirapine Regimen"; Adriana M. Campa et al., correspondence, "HIVNET Nevirapine Trials," *The Lancet*, November 20, 1999.

6: South Africa: Drug Trials and AIDS Denialism

1. Mannfred A. Hollinger, *Introduction to Pharmacology* (Philadelphia: Taylor & Francis, 1997), 9–10.

2. Audrey R. Chapman and Leonard S. Rubenstein, eds., *Human Rights and Health: The Legacy of Apartheid* (Washington, DC: American Association for the Advancement of Science, 1998), 17.

3. Samantha Power, "The AIDS Rebel," *New Yorker*, May 19, 2003, 54–67, 59.

4. Roy Porter, *The Greatest Benefit to Mankind: A Medical History of Humanity* (New York: W.W. Norton, 1997), 621.

5. Chapman and Rubenstein, eds., *Human Rights and Health*, 18–19, 43–54.

6. Ibid., 25–34, 40, 42, 109.

7. R.J. Biggar et al., "Regional Variation in Prevalence of Antibody Against Human T-Lymphotropic Virus Types I and III in Kenya, East Africa," *International Journal of Cancer*, June 15, 1985, 763–67.

8. Laurie Garrett, *The Coming Plague: Newly Emerging Diseases in a World Out of Balance* (New York: Penguin Books, 1994), 355–58.

9. Paul Farmer, *Infections and Inequalities: The Modern Plagues* (Los Angeles: University of California Press, 1999), 122.

10. Lawrence K. Altman, "Linking AIDS to Africa Provokes Bitter Debate," *New York Times*, November 21, 1985, A1.

11. Power, "The AIDS Rebel."

12. Interview with Costa Gazi, September 11, 2003.

13. Chris McGreal, "Dying for Drugs: South Africa's Sick Wait for Judgment Day: Multinationals Go to Court Today over a Law Aimed at Cutting the Cost of Medicines," *The Guardian*, March 5, 2001, 16.

14. Tom Cohen, "Claims of Breakthrough in AIDS Treatment Questioned," Associated Press, January 22, 1997; Power, "The AIDS Rebel."

15. "National Party Urges Sacking of Health Minister over AIDS Drug Issue," BBC Summary of World Broadcasts, February 7, 1997; Jack Lundin, "Nothing to Write Home About: Virodene," *Financial Mail* (South Africa), April 24, 1998.

16. Power, "The AIDS Rebel."

17. Chapman and Rubenstein, eds., *Human Rights and Health*, 78.

18. Interview with Costa Gazi, September 11, 2003; Power, "The AIDS Rebel."

19. The Anglo American program was plagued by delays and criticisms from union and AIDS activists. At first, workers feared the company would discriminate against them if they tested positive for HIV. "The mining industry has been very brutal and you can't expect confidence and trust that workers will not face dismissal if they test positive with HIV," said Welcome Mboniso, a miners union representative. Hundreds of workers die every year in mine accidents, he said. "It's already a killer industry." By 2005, Anglo American was providing free antiretroviral therapy to 2,000 of its employees in sub-Saharan Africa. Terry Macalister, "They Dare Not Speak Its Name," *The Guardian*, October 9, 2003; Lauren Mills, "Hope Amid an Appalling Epidemic," *Financial Times*, July 29, 2005; www.unaids.org/en/geographical+area/by+country/south+africa.asp.

20. "New Report Estimates HIV/AIDS Drug Market Will Triple in Value from $5 Billion in Annual Sales to $13 Billion in 2007," HIVandhepatitis.com, July 23, 2001.

21. Interview with Keymanthri Moodley, November 11, 2003.

22. Interview with Simon Yaxley, January 2002.

23. Interview with Caroline Loew, January 2002.

24. Penni Crabtree, "Tragedy Gave Boost to San Diego Biotech Firm's Push for Drug Approval," *San Diego Union-Tribune*, May 16, 2002.

25. "Hollis Eden Pharmaceuticals: Richard Hollis," *San Diego Magazine*, February 2001, 134.

26. Simon Barber, "US Aids Drug to Be Tested on SA Subjects," *Business Day*, October 2, 1998, 1.

27. John S. James, "HE2000 Begins Clinical Trials," *The Body*, June 4, 1999.

28. Crabtree, "Tragedy Gave Boost."

29. Public Citizen press release, "Company Loses Second Bid to Silence Stockholder Who Posted Critical Comments on Web," October 26, 2001.

30. Crabtree, "Tragedy Gave Boost."

31. Joseph Radford, "Combating HIV," *Corporate Africa*, Summer 2001.

32. Interview with Bob Marsella, September 10, 2003.

33. Hollis-Eden Pharmaceuticals Annual Report 2004, 4.

34. Interview with Keymanthri Moodley, November 11, 2003.

35. Andrew Pollack, "U.S. Approves New Once-a-Day AIDS Drug from Glaxo Rival," *New York Times*, July 3, 2003.

36. "Sixth Patient Dies in Suspended AIDS Trials," South African Press Association, April 23, 2000; "Might Be Impossible to Say if Nevirapine Killed 5 Women," South African Press Association, April 10, 2000; "Lack of AIDS Drugs for Poor Makes SA Ripe for Exploitation: Gazi," South African Press Association, April 24, 2000.

37. Interview with Costa Gazi, September 11, 2003.

38. "Sixth Patient Dies in Suspended AIDS Trials," South African Press Association; "Might Be Impossible to Say if Nevirapine Killed 5 Women," South African Press Association; "Lack of AIDS Drugs for Poor Makes SA Ripe for Exploitation," South African Press Association.

39. Ian Sanne et al., "Severe Hepatotoxicity Associated with Nevirapine Use in HIV-Infected Subjects," *Journal of Infectious Diseases*, March 15, 2005, 825–29.

40. Treatment Action Campaign press release, "MCC Decision to Deregister Nevirapine for Mother-to-Child Transmission Prevention Is Disturbing and Confusing," July 31, 2003.

41. Power, "The AIDS Rebel."

42. Mike Cohen, "South African Government Launches New Attack on Drug Companies," Associated Press, April 5, 2000.

43. "BI Offers Free Viramune to Developing Countries," *Pharma Marketletter*, July 7, 2000.

44. "Leave Them Be," *The Economist*, April 6, 2002.

45. Interview with Bob Marsella, September 19, 2003.

46. Adele Baleta, "South African Court Again Tells Government to Increase Access to AIDS Drug," *The Lancet*, March 30, 2002, 1132.

47. Interview with Jay Brooks Jackson, October 10, 2003.

48. The National Institute of Allergy and Infectious Diseases shut the site down and commenced a lengthy, fifteen-month-long audit. According to a review by NIAID, "certain aspects of the collection of primary data may not conform to FDA regulatory requirements." National Institute of Allergy and Infectious Diseases press release, "Review of HIVNET 012," March 22, 2002; National Institute of Allergy and Infectious Diseases Division of AIDS, *HIVNET 012 Monitoring Report*, March 2003, 10, 46, 49; John Solomon, "Top U.S. Officials Warned of Concerns Before AIDS Drug Sent to Africa," Associated Press, December 13, 2004.

49. Henry J. Kaiser Family Foundation, "South African Medicines Control Council Calls for Alternate Nevirapine Efficacy Data in 90 Days, Could Ban Use of Drug," August 1, 2003.

50. Treatment Action Campaign, "MCC Decision to Deregister Nevirapine"; "Nevirapine Deadline Extended to 6 Months," *Cape Argus*, September 16, 2003.

51. "Outrage as Medicines Control Council Rejects Results of Nevirapine Trials," South African Medical Association News, July 30, 2003.

52. "Manto Defends Herbal Research in the Fight Against Aids," South African Broadcasting Corporation, July 24, 2003.

53. Power, "The AIDS Rebel."

54. Jeremy Laurance, "The Bombay Copycats Who Sold Treatment for $1 a Day," *The Independent*, April 20, 2001, 17.

55. Robert Radtke, "India Must Steer a Middle Path on Generic Drugs," *Financial Times*, March 24, 2005, 13.

56. David Pilling, "Activists Jubilant in S Africa Drugs Case," *Financial Times*, April 20, 2001, 9.

57. "Government Makes Dramatic AIDS Pledge," *The Star*, August 7, 2003, 1. The battle to tackle AIDS in South Africa had hardly been won: according to a June 2005 World Health Organization

report, just 104,600 of more than 800,000 South Africans in need of antiretroviral therapy had access to it. See www.who.int/3by5/ support/june2005_zaf.pdf.

58. Donald G. McNeil, "Africans Outdo U.S. Patients in Following AIDS Therapy," *New York Times*, September 3, 2003, 1.

7: Outsourcing to India: The One Billion Body Politic

1. Alix M. Freedman, "Population Bomb: Two Americans Export Chemical Sterilizations to the Third World," *Wall Street Journal*, June 18, 1998, A1.

2. Sanjay Kumar, "Sterilization by Quinacrine Comes under Fire in India," *The Lancet*, May 17, 1997.

3. Laxmi Murthy, "Contraceptive Research: Need for a Paradigm Shift," *One India, One People*, July 2001, 18–20.

4. M.D. Gupte and D.K. Sampath, "Ethical Issues Considered in Tamil Nadu Leprosy Vaccine Trial," *Indian Journal of Medical Ethics*, January/March 2000.

5. Amit Sen Gupta, "Research on Hire," *Indian Journal of Medical Ethics*, October/December 2001.

6. Ganapati Mudur, "Johns Hopkins Admits Scientist Used Indian Patients as Guinea Pigs," *BMJ*, November 24, 2001, 1204.

7. Chandra Gulhati, "Illegal Trials on Letrozole: Hundreds of Women Used as Guinea Pigs," *Monthly Index of Medical Specialties India*, December 2003.

8. Jeetha D'Silva and Vikram Doctor, "Clinical Trials in Dock as Guinea Pigs Fail the Test," *Economic Times*, March 11, 2004.

9. Interview with Amar Jesani, November 25, 2003.

10. Shabnam Minwalla, "Many Doctors Rely on Skewed Data," *Times of India*, September 18, 2003.

11. "UN Raps India for Missing Literacy Deadline," *Hindustan Times*, November 9, 2005.

12. Ganapati Mudur, "Inadequate Regulations Undermine India's Health Care," *BMJ*, January 17, 2004, 124.

13. Manidipa Mukherjee, "In the Dock," *Humanscape*, March 1997, 29.

14. Interview with Amar Jesani, November 25, 2003.

15. P.K. Sarkar, "A Rational Drug Policy," *Indian Journal of Medical Ethics*, January/March 2004.

16. Nobhojit Roy, "Who Rules the Great Indian Drug Bazaar?" *Indian Journal of Medical Ethics*, January/March 2004.

17. Poornima Joshi, "The Cost of Falling Ill," *Hindustan Times*, March 18, 2001.

18. Monobina Gupta, "Tuberculosis Drugs Head Spurious List," *The Telegraph* (Calcutta), August 4, 2003.

19. Arindam Mukherjee, "Pills That Kill," *Outlook*, September 22, 2003, 52.

20. Daniel Pearl and Steve Stecklow, "Drug Firms' Incentives Fuel Abuse by Pharmacists," *Indian Express*, August 17, 2001, reprinted from *Wall Street Journal*.

21. Chandra Gulhati, "Irrational Fixed-Dose Combinations: A Sordid Story of Profits Before Patients," *Indian Journal of Medical Ethics*, January/March 2003.

22. Mukherjee, "Pills That Kill."

23. Chandra Gulhati, "Illegal, Unethical Promotion Hits New Highs," *Monthly Index of Medical Specialties India*, posted to e-drug list, April 1, 2004.

24. S.M. Moazzem Hossain, "Community Development and Its Impact on Health: South Asian Experience," *BMJ*, April 3, 2004, 830–31.

25. Anita K.M. Zaidi et al., "Burden of Infectious Diseases in South Asia," *BMJ*, April 3, 2004, 811.

26. Ganapati Mudur, "Hospitals in India Woo Foreign Patients," *BMJ*, June 5, 2004, 1338.

27. FDA News, "New Indian Patent Law Heralds Multinationals' Return," *Daily International Pharma Alert*, January 31, 2005.

28. FDA News, "Drug Majors Anticipate Final Approval for India's Patent Reform," *Daily International Pharma Alert*, January 25, 2005.

29. James Love, "Options to Traditional Patents," *Financial Express*, April 6, 2005.

30. Narayan Kulkarni, "The Trials Leader," *Biospectrum*, June 10, 2003.

31. Interview with Ken Getz, October 2003.

32. "Lifting India's Barriers to Clinical Trials," *CenterWatch*, August 2003, 1.

33. D'Silva and Doctor, "Clinical Trials in Dock."

34. Sandhya Srinivasan, "Discussion on Biomedical Research on Humans in India: A Short Review," Achutha Menon Centre for Health Science Studies and Sree Chitra Tirunal Institute for Medical Sciences and Technology, October 2000, 14.

35. D'Silva and Doctor, "Clinical Trials in Dock."

36. "Lifting India's Barriers to Clinical Trials," *CenterWatch*, 6.

37. Atul Gawande, "Dispatch from India," *New England Journal of Medicine*, December 18, 2003, 2383–86.

38. Interview with Nadeem Rais, November 25, 2003.

39. Reshma Patil and Toufiq Rashid, "Strong Medicine," *Sunday Express*, December 28, 2003, 11.

40. Gawande, "Dispatch from India."

41. Jayaprakash Narayan, "Healthcare Is Sick," *Humanscape*, September 2003, 17.

42. Interview with Yash Lokhandwala, November 28, 2003.

43. Madhumita Bose, "Doctor, Heal Thyself," *Business India*, June 24–July 7, 2002, 107.

44. Soma Wadha, "Hypocratic Practice," *Outlook*, February 3, 2003, 51.

45. Geoff Dyer, "Sepsis Treatment Makes Slow Start at Eli Lilly," *Financial Times*, March 5, 2002, 20.

46. Eli Lilly press release, "Lilly Launches World's Largest Severe Sepsis Clinical Trial: 11,000 Patients to Be Enrolled in Study of Xigris Use in Patients with Low Risk of Death," September 17, 2002.

47. "Eli Lilly Launches Xigris to Combat 'Blood Poisoning,'" *Business Line*, October 19, 2002.

48. Thomas M. Burton, "Left on the Shelf: Why Cheap Drugs That Appear to Halt Fatal Sepsis Go Unused—Steroids Need Big Human Trial, but Pharmaceutical Makers Lack Incentive to Fund One—Dr. Meduri's 15-Year-Quest," *Wall Street Journal*, May 17, 2002, A1.

49. Society of Critical Care Medicine, "ICU Issues and Answers: Sepsis: What You Should Know," available at www.sccm.org/patient_family_resources/support_brochure.

50. When the reaction causes blood pressure to drop, depriving organs of oxygen, it's called "septic shock." When the infection is in the bloodstream itself, it's called "septicemia." Eli Lilly

press release, "Lilly Launches World's Largest Severe Sepsis Clinical Trial"; Society of Critical Care Medicine, "ICU Issues and Answers."

51. Jane E. Brody, "New Hope for Taming Deadly Septic Shock," *New York Times*, March 5, 2002, F1.

52. Gina Kolata, "Halted at the Market's Door: How a $1 Billion Drug Failed," *New York Times*, February 12, 1993, A1; Sandra Sugawara, "FDA Test Concerns Send Centocor's Stock Plunging," *Washington Post*, April 16, 1992, B11.

53. E.J. Ziegler et al., "Treatment of Gram-Negative Bacteremia and Septic Shock with HA-1A Human Monoclonal Antibody Against Endotoxin. A Randomized, Double-Blind, Placebo-Controlled Trial," *New England Journal of Medicine*, February 14, 1991, 429–36.

54. Tim Friend, "Drug's Value 'Like Penicillin,'" *USA Today*, February 14, 1991, 1A.

55. Sandra Sugawara, "FDA Test Concerns Send Centocor's Stock Plunging," *Washington Post*, April 16, 1992, B11.

56. As Martin Tobin later pointed out, "If mortality is significantly decreased in one subgroup but overall mortality is not changed, logic dictates that some patients must have had an increased mortality." Martin J. Tobin, "The Role of a Journal in a Scientific Controversy," *American Journal of Respiratory and Critical Care Medicine* 168 (2003): 512.

57. Sally Squires, "Sepsis," *Washington Post*, October 1, 1991, Z11.

58. "Mortality rates in the patients without gram-negative bacteremia were as follows: placebo, 37% (292 of 793) and HA-1A, 41% (318 of 785)." If those on the drug had survived at the same rate as those on placebo, only 290 would have died rather than 318 (37 percent of 785). Richard V. McCloskey et al., "Treatment of Septic Shock with Human Monoclonal Antibody HA-1A," *Annals of Internal Medicine*, July 1, 1994, 1–5.

59. "Murphy to Up Stake," *New Orleans Times-Picayune*, January 19, 1993, C1.

60. "Drugmaker Takes a Nosedive," *Cleveland Plain Dealer*, January 19, 1993, 1F.

61. Kolata, "Halted at the Market's Door."

62. FDA Center for Drug Evaluation and Research, Anti-infective Drugs Advisory Committee, transcript, October 16, 2001, 12.

63. See www.vericc.org/o1_new/media_pbn_030908.htm.

64. Burton, "Left on the Shelf."

65. Ibid.

66. Gordon R. Bernard et al., "Efficacy and Safety of Recombinant Human Activated Protein C for Severe Sepsis," *New England Journal of Medicine*, March 8, 2001, 699–709.

67. Not to mention the fact that the steroid researchers had refused to let their placebo patients suffer for very long. After ten days, if patients hadn't responded, they were switched to the treated group. The move, while compassionate, could have muddied the results. Burton, "Left on the Shelf."

68. Bernard et al., "Efficacy and Safety of Recombinant Human Activated Protein C."

69. Ibid.

70. See content.nejm.org/early_release/.

71. " 'Sepsis: The Peril of Infection' a 'Cutting Edge Medical Report' iTV Special Premieres on the Health Network March 10," *PR Newswire*, March 8, 2001.

72. "Bayer to Form International Sepsis Forum," *Pharmaceutical Business News*, March 26, 1997.

73. According to the FDA analysis, there was but a one in twelve chance that this trend toward diminishing effectiveness and even harm had occurred simply by random chance. Bolstering the worrying trend was the fact that in unrelated studies sepsis researchers had similarly linked the severity of the disease with patients' responses to treatment, i.e. $P = .08$. FDA Center for Drug Evaluation and Research, Anti-infective drugs advisory committee, transcript, October 16, 2001.

74. FDA Center for Drug Evaluation and Research, Anti-infective Drugs Advisory Committee, 247; H. Shaw Warren et al., "Risks and Benefits of Activated Protein C Treatment for Severe Sepsis," *New England Journal of Medicine*, September 26, 2002, 1027–30.

75. Ibid.

76. Since the probability of the disturbing data on Xigris occurring by chance was higher than one out of twenty, neither the agency nor scientific convention required Lilly to mention it. The only hint emanating from the FDA was its statement that

"not everyone will benefit" from Xigris. FDA Center for Drug Evaluation and Research, Anti-infective Drugs Advisory Committee, 323; U.S. Food and Drug Administration press release, "FDA Approves First Biologic Treatment for Sepsis," November 21, 2001.

77. Jane E. Brody, "New Hope for Taming Deadly Septic Shock," *New York Times*, March 5, 2002, F7.

78. Burton, "Left on the Shelf."

79. Eli Lilly press release, "Lilly Launches World's Largest Severe Sepsis Clinical Trial."

80. Warren et al., "Risks and Benefits of Activated Protein C Treatment."

81. FDA Center for Drug Evaluation and Research, Anti-infective Drugs Advisory Committee, 263.

82. "Eli Lilly to Make India Sourcing Hub," *India Business World*, October 2002.

83. Eli Lilly press release, "Lilly Launches World's Largest Severe Sepsis Clinical Trial."

84. Interview with Farhad Kapadia, November 25, 2003.

85. Feroze Ahmed, "Parents Have the Heart to Let Them Die," *Hindu Online*, August 18, 2003.

86. Eli Lilly clinical trials Web site, at www.lillytrials.com.

87. John Wurzelmann, "Presentation on Eastern Europe," in Globalization of Clinical Trials panel, Maximizing Clinical Efficiency Phases conference (Washington, DC, October 9, 2003).

88. Edward Abraham, "Exploration of Drotrecogin Alfa (Activated) in Adult Patients with Severe Sepsis at Lower Risk of Death," presentation, American College of Chest Physicians annual meeting (Seattle, WA, October 2004).

89. Dante Landucci, "The Surviving Sepsis Guidelines: 'Lost in Translation,'" *Critical Care Medicine* 31, no. 7 (2004): 1598–99.

90. See www.esicm.org/PAGE_sursepsis/?1hmi.

91. Correspondence with D. Annane, February 2005.

92. P.C. Minneci et al., "Meta-Analysis: The Effect of Steroids on Survival and Shock During Sepsis Depends on the Dose," *Annals of Internal Medicine*, July 2004, 47–56.

93. "Eli Lilly Slashes Therapy Cost for Sepsis by 40 Pc," Global News Wire, July 31, 2004.

94. Greg S. Martin, "Ask the Experts about General Critical Care: Drotrecogin Alfa and Sepsis," Medscape from WebMD, posted September 1, 2004, on www.medscape.com/viewarticle/487221.

95. Andrew Pollack, "Viagra Shows Promise as Lung Therapy," *New York Times*, October 28, 2004, C8.

96. Abraham, "Exploration of Drotrecogin Alfa."

97. FDA Web site, *Medwatch*, February 11, 2005. Also, Xigris, "Postmarking Study Commitments," on www.accessdata.fda.gov.

98. See www.xigris.com.

99. Edward Abraham et al., "Drotrecogin Alfa (Activated) for Adults with Severe Sepsis and a Low Risk of Death," *New England Journal of Medicine*, September 29, 2005.

100. Alex Berenson, "Blockbuster Drugs Are So Last Century," *New York Times*, July 3, 2005.

101. "I don't have the actual details of the trial," he said. From correspondence with Dr. Farhad Kapadia, February 16, 2005.

8: Calibrating Ethical Codes

1. Interview with Ruth Faden, 2001.

2. David J. Rothman, "The Shame of Medical Research," *New York Review of Books*, November 30, 2000; Public Citizen, "Letter to the World Medical Association Expressing Alarm at the Current Draft Revised Version of the Declaration of Helsinki," HRG Publication #477, March 29, 1999.

3. Susan Okie, "Health Officials Debate Ethics of Placebo Use: Medical Researchers Say Guidelines Would Impair Some Studies," *Washington Post*, November 24, 2000, A3.

4. David Brown, "Medical Research Group Revises Guidelines on Placebos," *Washington Post*, October 8, 2000.

5. World Medical Association, "WMA History: Declaration of Helsinki," available at www.wma.net/e/history/helsinki.htm; World Medical Association, "Declaration of Helsinki: Ethical Principles for Medical Research Involving Human Subjects," available at www.wma.net; U.S. Food and Drug Administration, *Guidance for Industry: Acceptance of Foreign Clinical Studies*, March 2001, available at/www.fda.gov/cder/guidance/fstud.htm.

6. Brian Vastag, "Helsinki Discord? A Controversial Declaration," *JAMA*, December 20, 2000, 2984; Okie, "Health Officials Debate Ethics of Placebo Use."

7. FDA Division of Pulmonary and Allergy Drug Products, "Use of Placebo-Controls in Life Threatening Diseases: Is the Developing World the Answer?" *Scientific Rounds*, January 24, 2001.

8. Interview with Robert Temple, 2001.

9. U.S. Food and Drug Administration, *Guidance for Industry*.

10. E.M. Meslin, "Memorandum to the National Bioethics Advisory Commission. Materials Relating to Public Comments: International Report," November 21, 2000, cited in Public Citizen, "Letter to the National Bioethics Advisory Commission Criticizing Their Draft Report on Ethics of Research in Developing Countries," HRG Publication #1550, December 6, 2000, available at www.citizen.org/publications/release.cfm?ID=6751#N_2_.

11. Nancy Kass and Adnan A. Hyder, "Attitudes and Experiences of U.S. and Developing Country Investigators Regarding U.S. Human Subjects Regulation," commissioned paper, in National Bioethics Advisory Commission, *Ethical and Policy Issues in International Research: Clinical Trials in Developing Countries*, Washington, DC, May 2001.

12. A.A. Hyder et al., "Ethical Review of Health Research: A Perspective from Developing Country Researchers," *Journal of Medical Ethics*, February 2004, 68–72.

13. National Bioethics Advisory Commission, Recommendation 4.1 and 4.2, *Ethical and Policy Issues in International Research: Clinical Trials in Developing Countries*, April 2001, cited in WMA Workgroup, September 2003.

14. Okie, "Health Officials Debate Ethics of Placebo Use."

15. Bernhard Huitfeldt et al., "Choice of Control in Clinical Trials—Issues and Implications of ICH-E10," *Drug Information Journal*, October/December 2001, 1147–56.

16. "Declaration of Helsinki Placebo Rule Being Reconsidered," July 10, 2001, article provided by Dr. Ruth Macklin.

17. Interview with Delon Human, 2001.

18. See www.wma.net/e/policy/17-c_e.html.

19. Letter from Public Citizen to Delon Human, World Medical Association, August 28, 2003.

20. Laurence Hirsch and Harry Guess, "Some Clauses Will

Hinder Development of New Drugs and Vaccines," *BMJ* 323 (December 2001): 1417.

21. Pharmaceutical Research and Manufacturers Association discussion paper, June 2001, cited in World Medical Association, "Documentation for the Preparation of Note of Clarification on Paragraph 30 of the Revised Declaration of Helsinki," September 2003.

22. Some have interpreted the clarification to Paragraph 30 as an affirmation of the requirement that study drugs be provided after trials end. The clarification reads, "The WMA hereby reaffirms its position that it is necessary during the study planning process to identify post-trial access by study participants to prophylactic, diagnostic, and therapeutic procedures identified as beneficial in the study or access to other appropriate care. Post-trial access arrangements or other care must be described in the study protocol so the ethical review committee may consider such arrangements during its review." The ambiguity as to whether study drugs must be provided or must simply be identified and described to ethics committees "depends on what 'it' means," one bystander noted. See World Medical Association, "Workgroup Report on the Revision of Paragraph 30 of the Declaration of Helsinki," September 2003; World Medical Association, "Declaration of Helsinki," at www.wma.net; interview with Peter Lurie, March 22, 2005.

23. R.K. Lie et al., "The Standard of Care Debate: The Declaration of Helsinki Versus the International Consensus Opinion," *Journal of Medical Ethics* 30 (2004): 190–99.

24. Karen Palmore Beckerman, "Long-Term Findings of HIVNET 012: The Next Steps," *The Lancet*, September 13, 2003.

25. Interview with Jay Brooks Jackson, October 10, 2003.

26. S.H. Eshleman et al., "Selection and Fading of Resistance Mutations in Women and Infants Receiving Nevirapine to Prevent HIV-1 Vertical Transmission (HIVNET 012)," *AIDS* 15 (2001): 1951–57.

27. Beckerman, "Long-Term Findings of HIVNET 012."

28. "South Africa Ends Nevirapine Monotherapy in HIV PMTCT, Due to Resistance Issues," *Pharma Marketletter*, July 14, 2004.

29. "China Begins Legalizing Methadone as Part of Effort to Prevent HIV Transmission among Injection Drug Users," *Kaiser Daily HIV/AIDS Report*, August 12, 2004.

30. Anne Bennett Swingle, "The Pathologist Who Struck Gold," *Hopkins Medical News*, Spring/Summer 2001.

31. Interview with Jay Brooks Jackson, October 10, 2003.

32. Swingle, "The Pathologist Who Struck Gold."

33. Nadeeja Koralage, "China to Offer Free HIV Testing and Treatment," *BMJ*, April 24, 2004.

34. Letter from International AIDS Society to Secretary of the Expert Committee on the Selection and Use of Essential Medicines Policy, World Health Organization, January 14, 2005.

35. John G. McNeil et al., "HIV Vaccine Trial Justified," *Science*, February 13, 2004, 961.

36. Jon Cohen, "Disappointing Data Scuttle Plans for Large-Scale AIDS Vaccine Trial," *Science*, March 1, 2002, 1616.

37. "Thailand Going Through 3rd Phase of Developing AIDS Vaccine," *Global News Wire—Africa Asia Intelligence Wire*, February 28, 2005.

38. Richard Horton, "AIDS: The Elusive Vaccine," *New York Review of Books*, September 23, 2004.

39. Agence France Presse, "Experts Call for World's Largest HIV Vaccine Trial to Be Scrapped," Channel NewsAsia, July 15, 2004.

40. Interview with Robert Temple, September 2003.

9: The Emperor Has No Clothes: The Vagaries of Informed Consent

1. Interview with Sten Vermund, 2001; World Health Organization, *Control of Epidemic Menigococcal Disease: WHO Practical Guidelines*, 2d ed., 6–12.

2. World Health Organization, "Disease Outbreaks Reported: Meningococcal Meningitis in Nigeria," March 6, 1996.

3. Interview with Anne-Valerie Kaninda, 2001.

4. See FDA review, at www.fda.gov/cder/foi/nda/97/020760a .htm.

5. Interview with Anne-Valerie Kaninda, 2001; Roche Pharmaceuticals, "Rocephin (Ceftriaxone Sodium) for Injection" product information; Centers for Disease Control, "Meningococcal Disease Among College Students: ACIP Modifies Recommendations for Meningitis Vaccination," October 20, 1999.

6. World Health Organization, *Control of Epidemic Meningococcal Disease*, 22–23; correspondence with Maria Santamaria, 2001.

7. *Juan Walterspiel, MD v. Pfizer, Inc.*, Civil Action No. 3:98cv917, U.S. District Court, District of Connecticut, July 26, 1998, 3–4, 6, 9–10, 20; *Abdullahi v. Pfizer*, 51–52.

8. *Walterspiel, MD v. Pfizer, Inc.*, 10.

9. Ibid., 14.

10. Joe Stephens, "Where Profits and Lives Hang in Balance: Finding an Abundance of Subjects and Lack of Oversight Abroad, Big Drug Companies Test Offshore to Speed Products to Market," *Washington Post*, December 17, 2000, A1.

11. H. Veeken et al., "Priority During a Meningitis Epidemic: Vaccination or Treatment?" *Bulletin of the World Health Organization*, March 1998, 135.

12. Marie Doona and J. Bernard Walsh, "Use of Chloramphenicol as Topical Eye Medication: Time to Cry Halt? Bone Marrow Aplasia Also Occurs with Ocular Use," *BMJ*, May 13, 1995, 1217.

13. Stephens, "Where Profits and Lives Hang in Balance"; "Roche Unit's Drug Is Approved," *Wall Street Journal*, August 31, 1993, A4.

14. Nancy Kass and Adnan A. Hyder, "Attitudes and Experiences of U.S. and Developing Country Investigators Regarding U.S. Human Subjects Regulations," commissioned paper, National Bioethics Advisory Commission, *Ethical and Policy Issues in International Research: Clinical Trials in Developing Countries*, vol. 2, May 2001, B-9.

15. Ibid., B-5

16. Sharon LaFraniere et al., "The Dilemma: Submit or Suffer," *Washington Post*, December 19, 2000, A1.

17. P. Pitisuttithum et al., "Risk Behaviors and Comprehension among Intravenous Drug Users Volunteered for HIV Vaccine Trial," *Journal of the Medical Association of Thailand*, January 1997, 80.

18. Daniel W. Fitzgerald et al., "Comprehension During In-

formed Consent in a Less-Developed Country," *The Lancet*, October 26, 2002, 1301–2.

19. E. Hardy et al., *Informed Consent and Fertility Regulation in Brazil, Final Report*, 1998, unpublished, cited in Kass and Hyder, "Attitudes and Experiences," 48.

20. Q.A. Karim et al., "Informed Consent for HIV Testing in a South African Hospital: Is It Truly Informed and Truly Voluntary?" *American Journal of Public Health*, April 1, 1998, 637–40.

21. "South Africa: Rath Foundation Conduct Illegal Experiments," *Africa News*, September 5, 2005.

22. Niels Lynoe et al., "Obtaining Informed Consent in Bangladesh," *New England Journal of Medicine*, February 8, 2001, 460–61.

23. Kass and Hyder, "Attitudes and Experiences," B-28.

24. Ibid., B-27.

25. Mary Pat Flaherty et al., "Life by Luck of the Draw," *Washington Post*, December 22, 2000, A1.

26. East African Standard, "Kenya: Rarieda Guinea Pigs Insist They Were Tricked into Joining Study," *Africa News*, January 26, 2004.

27. Sergei Varshavsky, "Discover Russia for Conducting Clinical Research," *Applied Clinical Trials*, March 2002, 74–80.

28. "Jump Starting Clinical Trials in China," *CenterWatch*, July 2002.

29. Interview with Anne-Valerie Kaninda, 2001.

30. See, for example, Jared Diamond, *Guns, Germs, and Steel: The Fates of Human Societies* (New York: W.W. Norton, 1997), 117–22.

31. Daniel W. Fitzgerald et al., "Comprehension During Informed Consent in a Less-Developed Country," *The Lancet*, October 26, 2002, 1301–2.

32. National Bioethics Advisory Commission, *Ethical and Policy Issues in International Research: Clinical Trials in Developing Countries*, vol. 1, April 2001, 41.

33. Interview with Jonathan D. Moreno, March 22, 2005.

34. M. Upvall et al., "Negotiating the Informed-Consent Process in Developing Countries: A Comparison of Swaziland and Pakistan," *International Nursing Review* 48, no. 3 (2001): 188–92.

35. National Bioethics Advisory Commission, *Ethical and Policy Issues in International Research*, vol. 1, 48.

36. Kass and Hyder, "Attitudes and Experiences," B-27.

37. Ibid., B-28.

38. A.K. Sanwal et al., "Informed Consent in Indian Patients," *Journal of the Royal Society of Medicine*, April 1996, 196–98.

39. LaFraniere et al., "The Dilemma."

40. John C.M. Lee, "Clinical Research in China," *Drug Information Journal* 32 (1998): 1265S–73S.

41. Interview with Robert Temple, September 2003.

42. Pfizer correspondence with the *Washington Post* on Clinical Trials Series, available at www.pfizer.com/pfizerinc/about/press/trovanq&a.html.

43. Interview with Elaine Kusel, 2001.

44. Pfizer correspondence with the *Washington Post* on Clinical Trial Series; H. Veeken et al., "Priority During a Meningitis Epidemic: Vaccination or Treatment?" *Bulletin of the World Health Organization*, March 1998, 2.

45. Interview with Larry Baraff, 2001.

46. Interview with Solomon Benatar, November 10, 2003.

47. Joe Stephens, "Doctors Say Drug Trials' Approval Was Backdated," *Washington Post*, January 16, 2001, A1.

48. Pfizer correspondence with the *Washington Post* on Clinical Trial Series.

49. In the end, more than two hundred thousand Africans fell ill with meningitis, and despite the efforts of aid doctors who treated tens of thousands in Kano alone, twenty thousand died. Nobody would have known anything about the experiment in Kano had a *Washington Post* reporter not somehow gotten wind of it. The FDA later curtailed the use of Trovan when reports of liver damage surfaced. Joe Stephens, "Where Profits and Lives Hang in the Balance," *Washington Post*, December 17, 2000; Pfizer correspondence with the *Washington Post* on Clinical Trial Series.

50. Advisory Committee on Human Radiation Experiments, "History of Prison Research Regulation," *Final Report*, at tis.eh.doe.gov/ohre/roadmap/achre/chap9_4.html.

51. Daniel Moerman, *Meaning, Medicine, and the "Placebo Effect"* (Cambridge: Cambridge University Press, 2002), 128.

52. Advisory Committee on Human Radiation Experiments, "History of Prison Research Regulation," citing Stephen Gettinger and Kevin Krajick, "The Demise of Prison Medical Research," *Corrections Magazine*, December 1979, 12.

53. Neal Dickert and Christine Grady, "What's the Price of a Research Subject? Approaches to Payment for Research Participation," *New England Journal of Medicine*, July 15, 1999, 198–203.

54. Andrew Pollack, "In Drug Research, the Guinea Pigs of Choice Are, Well, Human," *New York Times*, August 4, 2004.

55. Interview with Ben Leff, August 25, 2003.

56. See www.indianabiblecollege.org/employment.htm.

57. See www.lillyclinic.com.

58. See www.lillyclinic.com/about/tour.htm.

59. "Test Subjects Call Lilly Screening Process Inadequate," Associated Press, March 4, 2004; Tom Murphy, "Clinical Trials Face Volunteer Challenges; Lilly Bucks National Trend, Reports No Enrollment Woes," *Indianapolis Business Journal*, July 19, 2004; "FDA Clears Lilly Drug in Suicide During Clinical Trial," Associated Press, August 12, 2004.

60. Elizabeth Shogren, "FDA Sat on Report Linking Suicide, Drugs," *Los Angeles Times*, April 6, 2004.

61. Deanna Wrenn, "Lilly Alters Procedure in Drug Test in Response to Suicide," Associated Press, March 5, 2004.

62. Carol Druga, "Woman Who Committed Suicide During Lilly Drug Study Was Trying to Earn Money for College," Associated Press, February 12, 2004.

63. "Participant in Drug Trial Found Dead of Suicide in Eli Lilly Lab," Associated Press, February 10, 2004.

64. "FDA Clears Lilly Drug in Suicide During Clinical Trial," Associated Press, August 12, 2004; Reuters, "Antidepressant by Eli Lilly Is Approved for Diabetics," *New York Times*, September 8, 2004; Shankar Vedantam, "Depression Drugs to Carry a Warning; FDA Orders Notice of Risks for Youths," *Washington Post*, October 16, 2004, A1; "Antidepressant Tied to Attempted Suicides," *New York Times*, July 2, 2005, 9.

65. Interview with Ben Leff, August 25, 2003.

66. Dickert and Grady, "What's the Price of a Research Subject?"

67. Department of Health and Human Services Office of Inspector General, *Recruiting Human Subjects: Pressures in Industry-Sponsored Clinical Research*, June 2000, 26.

68. Interview with Anamika Jithoo, November 2003.

69. Robert Helms, ed., *Guinea Pig Zero: An Anthology of the Journal for Human Research Subjects* (New Orleans, LA: Garrett County Press, 2002), 16.

70. Ibid., 40–43.

71. Department of Health and Human Services Office of Inspector General, *Recruiting Human Subjects*.

72. Ibid., 17.

73. Thomas Bodenheimer, "Uneasy Alliance—Clinical Investigators and the Pharmaceutical Industry," *New England Journal of Medicine*, May 18, 2000, 1539–44.

74. Department of Health and Human Services Office of Inspector General, *Recruiting Human Subjects*, 18.

75. Ibid.

76. Holcomb B. Noble, "Hailed as a Surgeon General, Koop Is Faulted on Web Ethics," *New York Times*, September 5, 1999, 1.

77. Nick Smith, "The Strains of Pharming It Out," *Scrip*, July/August 2002, 32.

78. Interview with Ken Getz, October 2003.

79. See www.threewire.com/Inside/About.htm.

80. See www.clinicalsolutionsonline.com/.

81. Robert Whitaker, "Lure of Riches Fuels Testing," *Boston Globe*, November 17, 1998.

82. Michael D. Lemonick and Andrew Goldstein, "At Your Own Risk: Some Patients Join Clinical Trials Out of Desperation, Others to Help Medicine Advance. Who Is to Blame if They Get Sick—Or Even Die?" *Time*, April 22, 2002.

83. National Bioethics Advisory Commission, *Ethical and Policy Issues in Research Involving Human Participants*, vol. 1, 3–4.

84. Lemonick and Goldstein, "At Your Own Risk."

85. Christopher K. Daugherty, "Impact of Therapeutic Research on Informed Consent and the Ethics of Clinical Trials: A Medical Oncology Perspective," *Journal of Clinical Oncology*, May 1999, 1601–17.

86. David F. Horrobin, "Are Large Clinical Trials in Rapidly

Lethal Diseases Usually Unethical?" *The Lancet*, February 22, 2003, 695–97.

87. Paul Root Wolpe, "Not Just How, but Whether: Revisiting Hans Jonas," *American Journal of Bioethics*, Fall 2003, vii–viii.

88. David A. Stone et al., "Patient Expectations in Placebo-Controlled Randomized Clinical Trials," *Journal of Evaluation in Clinical Practice* 11, no. 1 (2005): 77–84.

89. Franklin G. Miller and Donald L. Rosenstein, "The Therapeutic Orientation to Clinical Trials," *New England Journal of Medicine*, April 3, 2003, 1383–86.

90. Department of Health and Human Services Office of Inspector General, *Recruiting Human Subjects*.

91. Horrobin, "Are Large Clinical Trials in Rapidly Lethal Diseases Usually Unethical?"

92. Post on Breast Cancer Action Nova Scotia discussion group, at bca.ns.ca/indice/2003/65index.cgi/noframes/read/249686.

93. Moerman, *Meaning, Medicine, and the "Placebo Effect,"* 105–6.

94. Ibid., 41.

95. Interview with Dr. Farhad Kapadia, November 29, 2003.

96. "The Use of Innovative Strategies in Patient Recruitment: Best Practices and Success Stories from Pharma and Biotech," panel discussion, Maximizing Clinical Efficiency Phases, Washington, DC, October 8–10, 2003.

97. Interview with Larry J. Baraff, January 10, 2002.

98. Robert I. Misbin, "Placebo-Controlled Trials in Type 2 Diabetes," *Diabetes Care* 24, no. 4 (2001): 768–74.

99. Interview with Jonathan D. Moreno, March 22, 2005.

100. Adrian Michaels, "Pfizer Suit Adds to Pressure on Industry," *Financial Times*, September 3, 2001, 8; Reuters, "Case over Pfizer Clinical Trial in Nigeria Is Reopened," *New York Times*, October 14, 2003, 4.

10: Tipping the Scales

1. Anne Bennett Swingle, "The Pathologist Who Struck Gold," *Hopkins Medical News*, Spring/Summer 2001.

2. "President Nixon, you can cure cancer," philanthropist Mary Lasker and her allies boldly claimed in a *New York Times* advertisement. "We lack only the will and the kind of money . . . that went into putting a man on the moon." Gary Cohen and Shannon Brownlee, "Mary and Her 'Little Lambs' Launch a War," *U.S. News & World Report*, February 5, 1996, 76; U.S. Bureau of Census, "Deaths by Major Causes: 1960 to 2001," *Statistical Abstract of the United States, 2003*, Washington, DC, January 2003, 91.

3. Roy Porter, *The Greatest Benefit to Mankind: A Medical History of Humanity* (New York: W.W. Norton, 1997), 580.

4. Abigail Trafford, "Fanfare Fades in the Fight Against Cancer," *U.S. News & World Report*, June 19, 1978, 63.

5. Interview with Ruth Faden, 2001.

6. Anne-Emannuelle Bim, "Gates' Grandest Challenge: Transcending Technology as Public Health Ideology," *The Lancet*, March 11, 2005.

7. Interview with Dr. Solomon Benatar, November 10, 2003.

8. FDA News, "CDC Revises Guidelines for Expanded Use of Preventive HIV Regimens," *Drug Daily Bulletin*, January 31, 2005.

9. Sabin Russell, "Antiviral Drug Used to Treat AIDS to Be Tested as Vaccine," *San Francisco Chronicle*, December 1, 2004.

10. National Center for HIV, STD, and TB Prevention, Divisions of HIV/AIDS Prevention, *CDC Trials of Daily Oral Tenofovir for Preventing HIV Infection*, Centers for Disease Control, February 17, 2005.

11. Ibid.

12. "Daily Tenofovir DF to Prevent HIV Infection among Sex Workers in Cambodia," clinical trial listing, clinicaltrials.gov.

13. Family Health International, "FHI Oral Tenofovir Study," available at www.fhi.org.

14. Human Rights Watch, *Not Enough Graves: Thailand's War on Drugs, HIV/AIDS and Violations of Human Rights*, July 2004, cited in Thai AIDS Treatment Action Group et al. press release, "Thai Activists Speak Out on Tenofovir Trial in IDUs," December 8, 2004, and "Thailand's 'War on Drugs' Had Unexpected Consequences, New Study Says," Associated Press, March 30, 2005.

15. Sabin Russell, "Prostitutes Protest AIDS-Drug Test, Bay Area Company Hit with Charges of Exploitation," *San Francisco Chronicle*, July 14, 2004; Marilyn Chase and Guatam Naik, "Key AIDS Study in Cambodia Now in Jeopardy," *Wall Street Journal*, August 12, 2004, B1.

16. ACT UP Paris and Asian Pacific Network of Sex Workers press release, "Gilead Organizes the Infection of Sex Workers," July 15, 2004.

17. Chase and Naik, "Key AIDS Study in Cambodia."

18. "Cambodia's Premier Halts Planned Trials of AIDS Drug," Associated Press, August 11, 2004.

19. Thai AIDS Treatment Action Group et al. press release, "Thai Activists Speak Out on Tenofovir Trials in IDUs."

20. ACT UP Paris press release, "The Cameroonian Government Must Condemn Unethical Trials, and Not People Living with HIV/AIDS," January 25, 2005.

21. Jon Cohen, "Cameroon Suspends AIDS Study," *Science*, February 4, 2005.

22. Andrew Jack and Michael Peel, "AIDS Study Runs into Trouble in Nigeria," *Financial Times*, March 15, 2005, 12.

23. Cohen, "Cameroon Suspends AIDS Study."

24. "A Public Statement from the Global Campaign for Microbicides and the AIDS Vaccine Advocacy Coalition on the Impact of Stopping Tenofovir Trials in Cambodia and Cameroon," February 18, 2005.

25. Chase and Naik, "Key AIDS Study in Cambodia."

26. Andrew Jack, "Mission to Save AIDS Drug Trial from Ethical Whirlpool," *Financial Times*, February 23, 2005, 24.

27. Interview with Mitchell Warren, March 24, 2005.

28. Cohen, "Cameroon Suspends AIDS Study."

29. Sabin Russell, "Prostitutes Protest AIDS-Drug Test."

30. Center for HIV Identification, Prevention, and Treatment Services, "Anticipating the Efficacy of HIV Preexposure Prophylaxis (PrEP) and the Needs of At-Risk Californians," November 2004.

31. Shambavi Subbarao et al., "Chemoprophylaxis with Oral Tenofovir Disoproxil Fumarate (TDF) Delays but Does Not Prevent Infection in Rhesus Macaques Given Repeated Rectal Chal-

lenges of SHIV," Conference on Retroviruses and Opportunistic Infections, Boston, February 22–25, 2005.

32. AIDS Vaccine Advocacy Coalition, "Will a Pill a Day Prevent HIV? Anticipating the Results of the Tenofovir 'PREP' Trials," March 2005, 1.

33. Interview with John Wurzlemann, October 9, 2003.

34. Interview with Jay Brooks Jackson, October 10, 2003.

35. Seth Berkley, "Thorny Issues in the Ethics of AIDS Vaccine Trials," *The Lancet*, September 20, 2003, 992.

36. Interview with Nadeem Rais, November 25, 2003.

37. TROUT Review Group, "How Do the Outcomes of Patients Treated with Randomized Control Trials Compare with Those of Similar Patients Treated Outside These Trials?" available at hiru.mcmaster.ca/ebm/trout.

38. Interview with Arthur Ammann, 2001.

39. Interview with Macé Schuurmans, November 13, 2003.

40. Pfizer correspondence with the *Washington Post* on Clinical Trials Series, available at www.pfizer.com/pfizerinc/about/press/trovanq&a.html.

41. Joe Stephens, "Where Profits and Lives Hang in Balance: Finding an Abundance of Subjects and Lack of Oversight Abroad, Big Drug Companies Test Offshore to Speed Products to Market," *Washington Post*, December 17, 2000.

42. Interview with Macé Schuurmans, November 13, 2003.

43. Interview with Yash Lokhandwala, November 28, 2003.

44. E-mail correspondence with Mary Ngoma, January 24, 2005.

45. Interview with Yash Lokhandwala, November 28, 2003.

46. Interview with Solomon Benatar, November 11, 2003.

47. Interview with Leslie London, November 11, 2003.

Conclusion

1. Interview with Solomon Benatar, November 11, 2003.

Acknowledgments

Thanks first to Mark, Zakir, and Kush Bulmer, who supported me throughout the writing of this book. Hasmukh Shah, MD; Hansa Shah, MD; David Bulmer, MD; and Carolyn Bulmer provided much-needed encouragement and translation. Peter Lurie, MD; Anthony Arnove; Andy Hsiao; Esther Kaplan; and Gregg Weinberg, among others, helped develop the ideas in this book. Grateful thanks also to Gita and Babulin Shah in Mumbai and to Martin and Jessica McEwan in South Africa, as well as the many clinicians, investigators, ethicists, activists, and patients who shared their stories with me.

Index

235